37 LIFE LESSONS LEARNED ON A BIKE TRIP ACROSS THE UNITED STATES

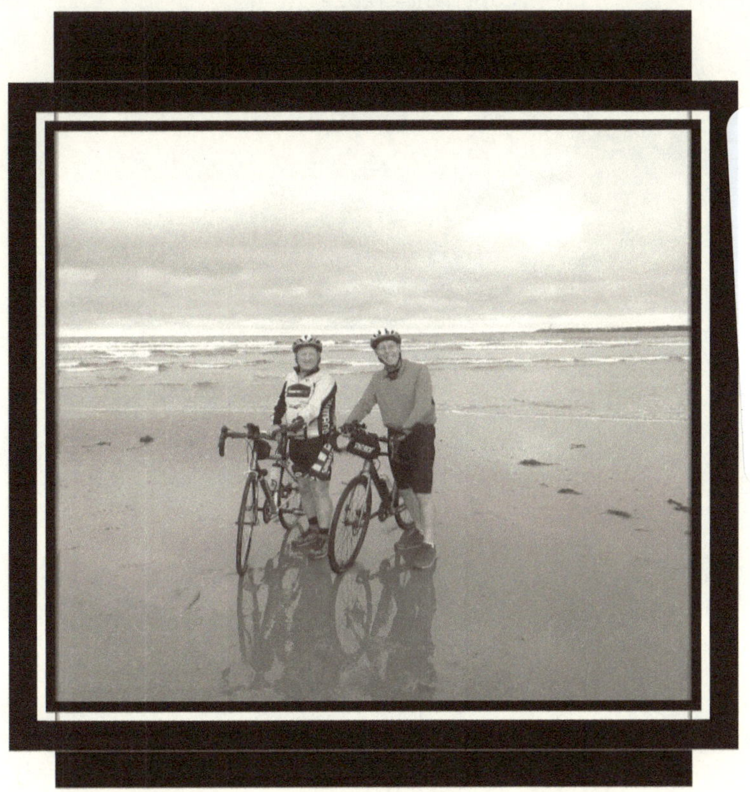

By JOHN RAYMOND

Contents

Dedication...1

INTRODUCTION...3

START OF TRIP...7

On April 9, 2022 7

April 10, 2022- Day 2..9

April 11, 2022 – Day 3 11

April 12, 2022-Day 4 13

April 13, 2022-Day 5 15

April 14, 2022-Day 6 17

April 15, 2022-Day 7 19

April 16, 2022 - Day 8..21

April 17, 2022-Day 9 23

April 18, 2022 – Day 2 of the Bike Ride......................26

April 19, 2022 – Day 3 of the Bike Ride......................29

April 20, 2022 – Day 4 of the Bike Ride......................32

April 21, 2022 – Day 5 of the Bike Ride......................35

April 22, 2022 – Day 6 of the Bike Ride......................38

April 23, 2022 – Day 7 of the Bike Ride..................................41

April 24, 2022 – Day 8 of the Bike Ride..................................44

April 25, 2022 - Day 9 of the Bike Ride 47

April 26, 2022 – Day 10 of the Birke Ride 50

April 27, 2022 – Day 11 of the Bike Ride................................53

April 28, 2022 – Day 12 of the Bike Ride................................56

April 29, 2022 – Day 13 of the Bike Ride................................59

April 30, 2022 – Day 14 of the Bike Ride................................62

May 1, 2022 - Day 15 of the Bike Ride 64

May 2, 2022 - Day 16 of the Bike Ride 67

May 3, 2022 – Day 17 of the Bike Ride 69

May 5, 2022 – Day 19 of the Bike Ride 76

May 6, 2022 – Day 20 of the Bike Ride 80

May 7, 2022 – Day 21 of the Bike Ride 82

May 8, 2022 - Day 22 of the Bike Ride 87

May 9, 2022 – Day 23 of the Bike Ride 91

May 10, 2022 – Day 24 of the Bike Ride 93

May 11, 2022 – Day 25 of the Bike Ride 96

May 12, 2022 – Day 26 of the Bike Ride 99

About the Book..105

Dedication

My Children: Lura and Tony, as well as all of my future Grandchildren (presently Teddy and George). You are my motivators and the main reason for making this Bike Trip. You can do anything you want in life if you put your mind, body and soul into your goals.

As my wife Joleen once told me, "Hold Close Your Dreams!"

INTRODUCTION

Many people ask, "Why would you want to do this long enduring Bike Trip?" "Wouldn't it be easier just to ride the route in your camper?"

This is a very common question, and I can only answer it from my perspective:

1. It has been a dream of mine since my late-twenties to complete a bike trip across the United States. Accomplishing this trip fulfills a personal goal that I have had for decades. Now that family and work responsibilities are decreased, it is time to accomplish this "bucket list" task.

2. My main motivator for making this trip was for my children and grandchildren.
   The message to them: You can do anything you want if you put your mind, body and soul into your goals in life. Hold Close Your Dreams!

3. We did this trip in memory of our lost family members. For Phil, it was his brother, Guy. For me, it was my wife, Joleen. Both died of cancer. As we rode and sometimes were tired and sore, we thought of them and how they suffered much more than us. This kept us motivated. As

part of our ride, we were able to raise over $1300 in donations for the American Cancer Society.

4. Send a message to my patients who struggle with addictions to tobacco, alcohol and drugs. You can accomplish anything if you put your mind to it!

5. For anyone considering live organ donation but fearing it will affect their physical activity. I was a kidney donor to my brother Paul in 2013. Fortunately, everything went well, and he is living a normal life again after being on dialysis for a year.

    The message: You can do amazing physical work after being a live organ donor. Don't hesitate. Give the gift of life!

6. On the trip, there was much time to reflect on our lives: What you've accomplished, where you are presently, and what you hope to achieve in the future. We are blessed to have been given the gift of good health. We all have a purpose for being on this Earth. Let's make the most of this opportunity!

7. Finally, this trip has brought us closer to God. His creation is amazing! His gift of life is a blessing! Let us all be thankful.

37 Life Lessons Learned On A Bike Trip Across The United States

Have you ever had something you wanted to accomplish in your life but weren't sure if it would ever happen? Many of us have gone through this process of keeping a "bucket list" updated. However, as we age, some of these items become more difficult, if not impossible, to occur.

Since the age of 28, one of my goals items in life was to complete a bicycle trip across the United States. However, many life events prevented this from occurring. Between family obligations and work schedules, the thought of going across the country on a bike was put on the "back burner." Now that the children are grown and have started their own families and work retirement is here, this was an ideal opportunity to achieve that goal – even at the age of 65. With the help and support of a good high school friend, Phil Roy, who is also a very active cyclist, we planned out our adventure. After two years of planning during the COVID pandemic, we set a date for April 2022 to embark on our adventure across the United States.

The following is a daily Journal of our trip. Our initial goal was to be physically healthy enough to complete the journey. We also wanted to "see the world" and visit many of the sites in the southern United States.

As we started the trip, we discovered that we were experiencing much more than our original goal. The trip became more of a Pilgrimage. Each day brought new experiences relating to basic life lessons. These lessons are explained at the center of each daily journal entry. As you will see, specific experiences occurred each day that reflected on the important things we often take for granted in life. The trip reminded us of what's important in life so we can pass it on to our children and grandchildren. It allowed us time to reflect on where we've been with our lives, where we presently stand, and what we want to accomplish for the rest of our lives. It also allowed us to see the country in a very different way and to appreciate her beauty. We also grew closer to God as we observed the beauty of His creation and how He reached out and touched us on this trip.

So let me share our story...

START OF TRIP

On April 9, 2022

Phil and I met in Bangor, Maine, to start our journey. Our destination was to drive the RV camper to San Diego, where we would start our bike trip, going west to east. We loaded up our bikes into a 22-foot RV and started our journey down the State of Maine. There was still snow in Northern Maine; however, the Bangor area had no snow but had signs of early spring which we call "mud season."

Our first stop was in Portland, Maine, where we met up with Phil's sister, Terry, for lunch at a local sub shop. It was great to see her again since COVID had limited our visitations the last two years. After lunch, we continued driving down Interstate 95, switching to Interstate 495 and heading toward Connecticut.

On the way, we were able to meet up with my son, Tony and his girlfriend, Megan, in Boxboro, Massachusetts. It was great to see them! They brought gifts for our trip that included a notepad, a deck of cards, lip balm, and a special card wishing us luck on our trip. They also provided a box of granola bars, which are my favorite!

After our meeting, we proceeded down to Connecticut, where we met up with Phil's other sister Mariette and her husband, Guy, who were terrific hosts at their wonderful home in Newington, Connecticut. We stayed there our first night. Phil stayed up late that night with his sister reminiscing about the past.

Today's Lesson: Family is everything. We may meet many friends in our lives. But family love and support is incomparable!

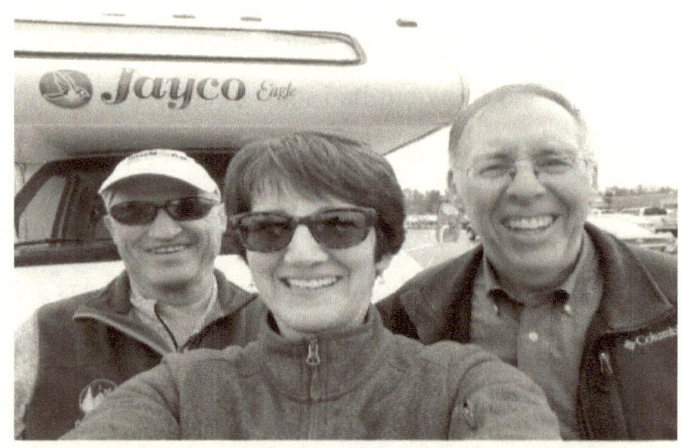

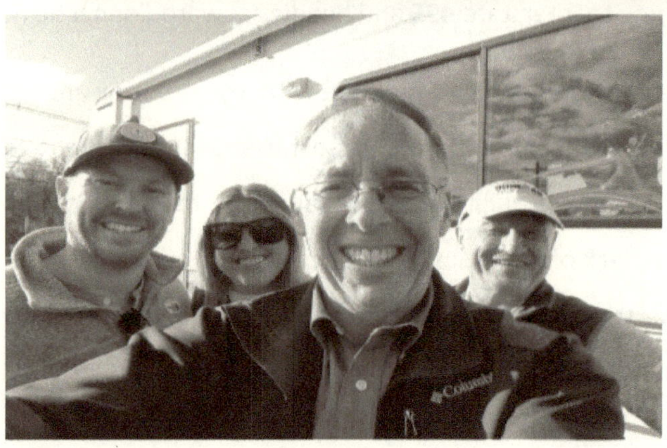

April 10, 2022- Day 2

Our day started early by rearranging and repacking the RV, filling up the water tank, and starting our journey toward Pennsylvania. Our original plan was to bypass New York City by taking Interstate 84 through Connecticut. However, our GPS took us through a different route straight towards NYC! Wanting to avoid the George Washington Bridge, we quickly took Route 87 around the City of New York, over the Mario Como Bridge (Tappan Zee Bridge) into White Plains, New York. It was there that we met the worst roads on our trip.

There were many potholes and crevasses throughout the road. There, we noticed many rattles coming from the RV walls and significant vibration from the front end of the vehicle. Despite this, we continued to Columbia, Pennsylvania, to meet with Phil's son and wife, Dan and Hannah. We were greeted with a warm welcome into their brand-new home that they had purchased only a few months prior. After a grand home tour, we headed for a wonderful meal at a local restaurant.

On the way back home, Dan and Hannah were sitting in the front seats, holding hands and not saying a word. Love was present. It reminds me of the days of starting a family and sharing the love with my wife. We returned back to their house to continue conversations while watching a baseball game on

TV. It was great to see them as they are expecting their first child in 3 months!

Today's Lesson: Love with a spouse is precious. Do not take it for granted!

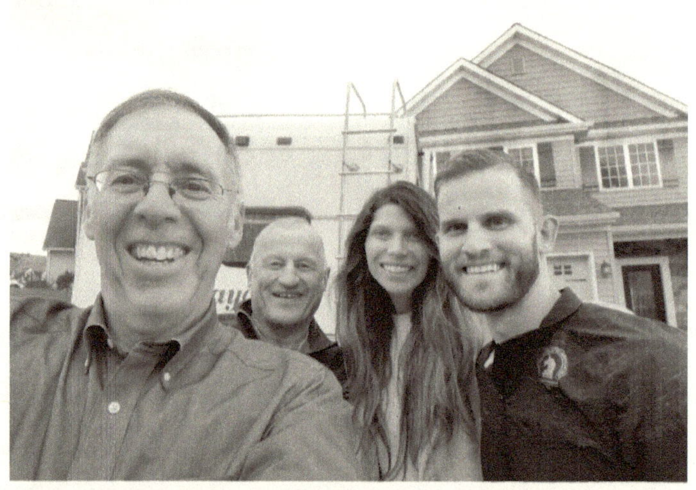

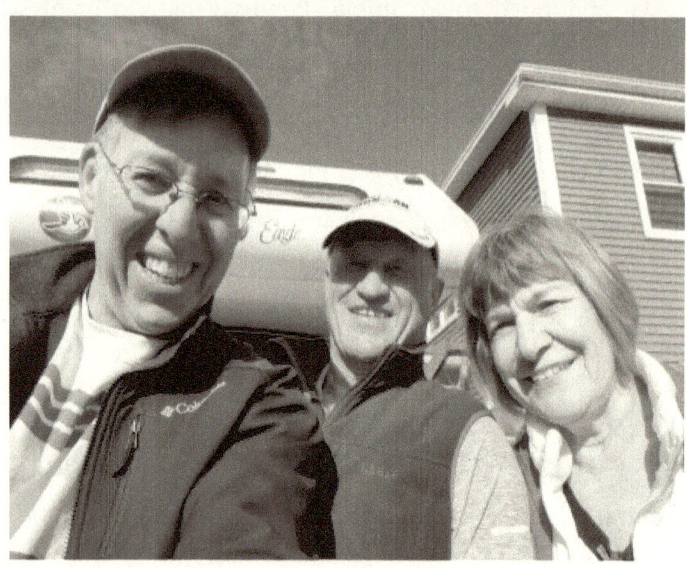

April 11, 2022 – Day 3

The day started with concern for the front tires on the RV. After checking the passenger's side tire, it was noted to have significant wear. We also noted a lost hubcap on the right rear wheel. We suspected that the terrible roads around New York City were to blame.

After a few calls, we were fortunate to locate a wonderful garage that took us right in to change the front tires. We met the Manager who was curious about our reason for travel. He shared with us that years ago, he also accomplished a bucket list item by traveling 1500 miles on his motorcycle in 24 hours, joining an elite national club. His wife thought he was crazy, "and maybe she was right." He shared this with a smile and pride, noting that he couldn't do it again at his present age. However, the memory was still vivid in his mind.

With new tires and an oil change on the RV, we noticed a difference in the driving control immediately. We left Harrisburg, Pennsylvania heading South on Route 81. The landscape was beautiful as spring had arrived in the Blue Ridge Mountains. A string of purple blossoms lined the sides of the road, while the hardwoods in the hills were dark green in color. The new grass in the cattle farms was emerald green as cows grazed. By nightfall, we made it to Fall Branch, Tennessee, just outside Johnson City, where we parked at a local Walmart for the night. We restocked our supplies and settled for the night.

Today's Lesson: Hold on to your dreams. People may think you are crazy with your bucket list, but for you, nothing is more important.

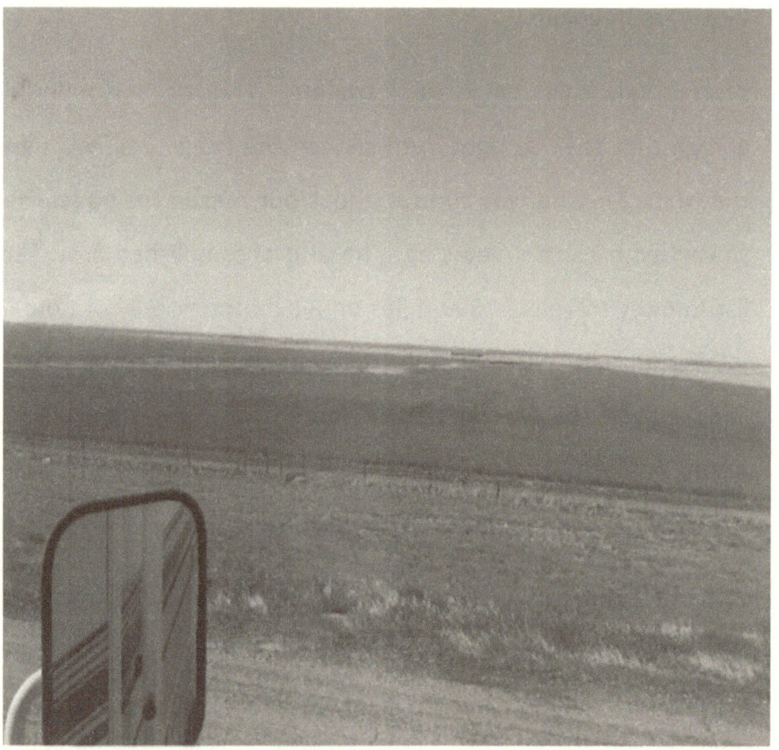

April 12, 2022-Day 4

We had an early jump on our driving expedition this morning, starting at 06:15 am. We immediately ran into some very heavy rain that lasted most of the morning.

Our day started in Branch Fall, Tennessee, driving down Interstate 40 West through the Smoky Mountains. Now we know why they are called the Smoky Mountains since it looks like there is always smoke in the hills, especially on a rainy day. We went by Knoxville, Tennessee and then headed toward Nashville. After numerous calls to RV centers as well as Ford dealerships looking for a hubcap to replace the one we had lost, we ended up at a very small auto repair shop where we were met by a wonderful Middle Eastern gentleman who was very willing to help us.

His brother soon arrived and started a conversation with us. Phil was anxious to tell him about our planned trip. He was proud to tell him that he was from Northern Maine, at which time the brother asked, "Where is Maine?" Phil replied, "it's in New England, at which time the brother said, "Is that in California?" We did not know what else to say! The mechanic was able to fix the wheel, and we were on our way. Our trip continued through Nashville, a very beautiful city that seems worth revisiting at length someday. The Nashville skyline was beautiful! We continued our journey on Interstate 40 West. By now, the sky had cleared, and the driving was easier. However, we drove into some significant construction as we approached Memphis, Tennessee, the last stop before the Mississippi River. We followed the map north of Memphis and crossed a huge bridge that goes across the Mississippi River. We later researched the internet and found that the bridge was 1 mile long! After the bridge, we were now in Arkansas, which was a surprise to us. The section between the Mississippi River and Little Rock, Arkansas, was mostly large farmlands and very flat. We continued to a KOA campground north of Little Rock, Arkansas, where we stayed for the night after a Papa John's pizza. It was a long day of driving (nearly 12 hours and over 620 miles).

Today's lesson: Be proud of where you're from, and do not be embarrassed to tell people about your homeland.

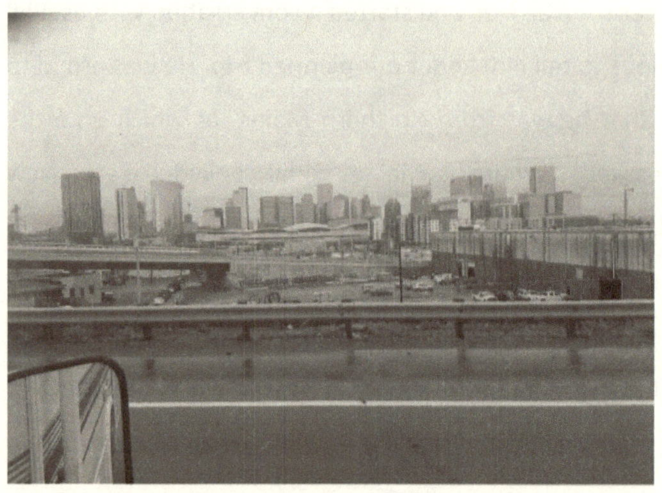

April 13, 2022-Day 5

The day started early, around 6:30 am. We were on the road heading west on Interstate 40. Approximately 50 miles down the road, we listened to a local radio station announcing heavy storms heading our way. They were reporting winds of 50 miles an hour, with tornado warnings announced by the meteorologist. The storm was approximately 30 miles ahead of where we were driving. Because of this, we pulled into a local Walmart parking lot and waited for the storm to pass. We could hear the heavy rain falling while we were safely shopping in Walmart. It took approximately 3 hours for the storm to pass.

Once it was safe, we departed Arkansas and onto Oklahoma. We were amazed at the flatness of the landscape and how few towns we saw until we reached Oklahoma City. We were impressed by the beauty of Oklahoma City and its skyline. We continued into western Oklahoma, where we settled at a Walmart parking lot in Elk City, Oklahoma, which is known as the mid-way point in the United States. We had a nice meal at a family restaurant and later settled down for the evening.

Today's lesson: Make sure to be safe when you see danger ahead. It is okay to stop and wait until the danger passes.

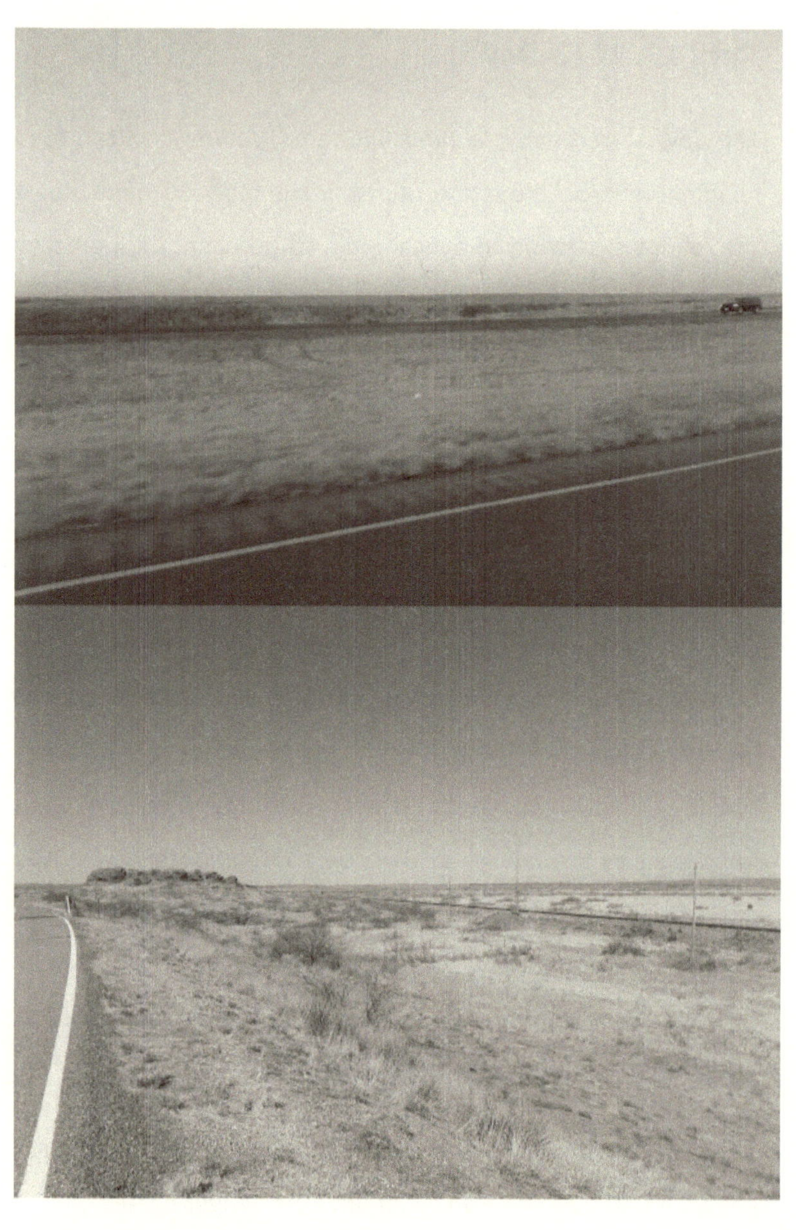

April 14, 2022-Day 6

We left Oklahoma in the early part of the day. As soon as we crossed into the northern section of Texas, we immediately saw many windmills - hundreds of them on both sides of the road as far as we could see! These were large windmills located in deserted fields with occasional farmlands.

This scenery continued for miles until we reached Amarillo, Texas. For a State that is known for oil fields, Texas definitely has changed its approach to power generation. We continued past northern Texas into New Mexico, where we saw a whole new landscape of dry grass and parched fields in the Northern plains. It looked like an area that had been under a drought for years!

This landscape continued for many miles until we reached Albuquerque, New Mexico. As we approached Albuquerque, we experienced a modern-looking city that seemed to have much to offer. We took a quick break to stretch our legs and rest the camper engine. Gaining some energy, we continued through the rest of New Mexico and into eastern Arizona. This area had rare organized farms and many dry, parched upper plains that expanded forever!

At the end of these deserted fields, in the far distance, were large mountain ranges that you would expect to see in textbook pictures of the west. We continued through Winslow, Arizona, where we had to sing "Take it Easy" by the Eagles. After a long day of traveling over 750 miles and 12 hours of driving, we settled in Flagstaff, Arizona, exhausted. We stayed at a campground that night. The morning temperature was 35°.

Today's lesson: New sources of energy must be refined, such as wind power, to save this planet from the pollution of fossil fuels. Let us all be good to our beautiful planet!

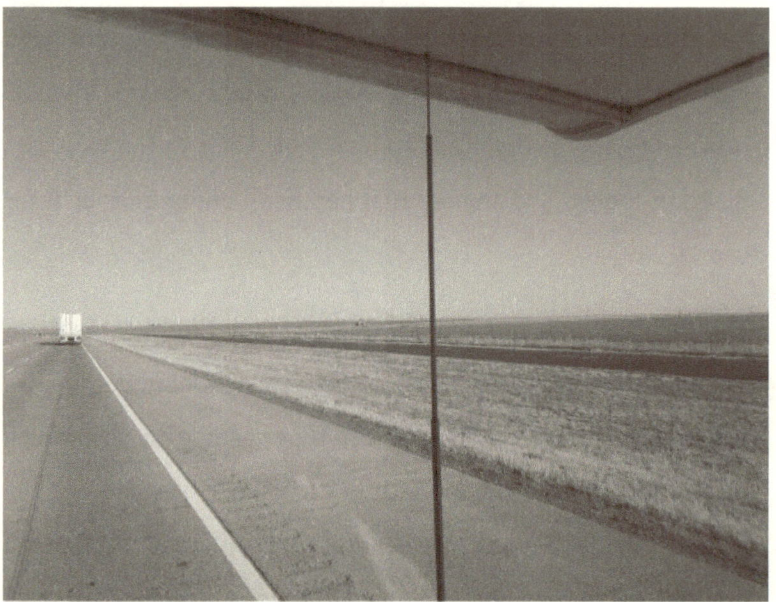

April 15, 2022-Day 7

We decided to take a detour from the highway and visit the South Rim of the Grand Canyon. This was a 3-hour detour, but was very much worth it. The Grand Canyon is gorgeous and breathtaking! We followed a walking trail around the rim, taking many pictures of the beauty. We learned much about the formation of the Canyon, made by the Colorado River, starting 450 million years ago! If you get the chance to visit the Grand Canyon, please do. It's incredibly beautiful!

Leaving the Grand Canyon, we took Route 180, returning to Flagstaff. On the way, we saw some very impoverished areas with very small homes in some Native American townships. How could poverty be so prevalent in such a beautiful area?

We continued down to Flagstaff, dropping from an elevation of over 8000 feet to approximately 7000 feet. Leaving Flagstaff, we took Route 17 South toward Phoenix, Arizona. The sites were exactly what we expected of the Arizona deserts, with large cactus plants and surrounding mountains.

By the time we reached Phoenix, we had dropped from an elevation of 7000 feet down to sea level. We drove around Phoenix and ended up in Calexico, California, for the night at a local Walmart parking lot. We were located just a few miles from the Mexican border. It was a long day of travel, and we were very tired from driving!

Today's lesson: Sometimes, we have to go through poverty and suffering in order to reach life's beauty. Be persistent with your goals!

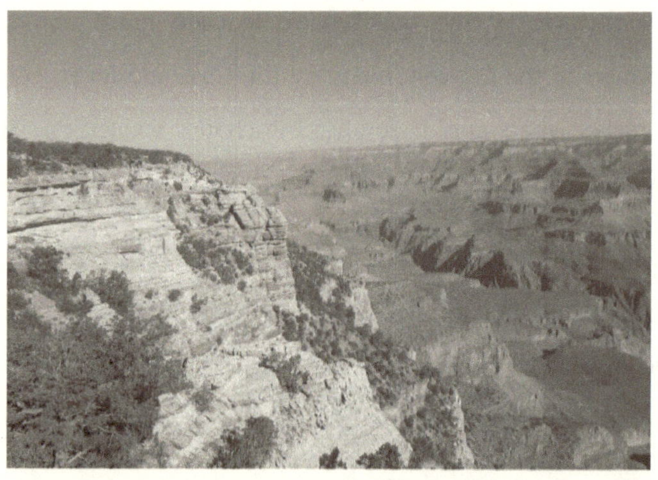

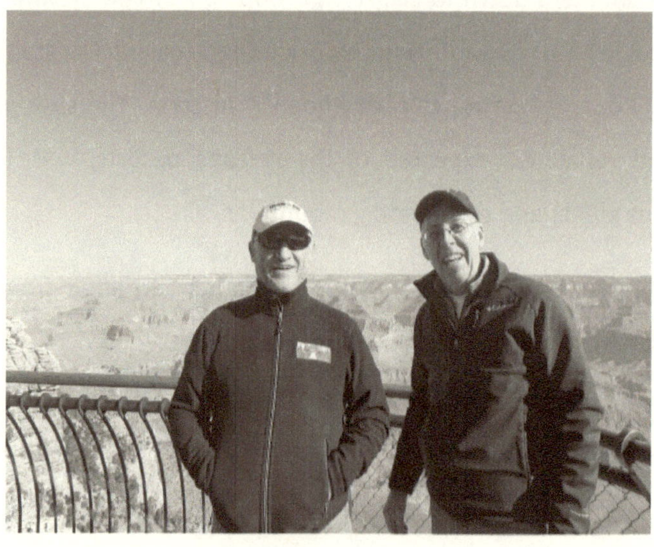

April 16, 2022 - Day 8

We took off from Calexico, California, early in the morning. The first stop was a gas station where Phil was frustrated with the attendant who could not get the gas pumps to work. Phil was trying to be courteous, but the attendant did not know how to work the pumps and was not able to help. He stated, "I do not know how to do this." So we left the gas station without getting gas and continued down the street to a second gas station to fill up our tank.

We went back on Interstate 8, heading towards San Diego. We started in desert areas but soon found ourselves climbing above a large mountain range in western California. It was an incredible climb! Bella (La Belle), our new name for the camper, did very well across some incredible elevations. The mountains that we climbed looked like rock piles, with large boulders making up the mountains. We finally arrived at our destination, San Diego, California, where our first stop was Balboa Park. It is a very large area in San Diego that contains many shops, museums and even the San Diego Zoo.

We decided to walk around the area to experience the street shows and entertainment. We also visited the air museum, where we found many unique plane replicas. We then drove near the shores of San Diego, ending up in the Torrey Pines area. The city of San Diego is beautiful and worth visiting. We then headed to our campsite in Julie Vista, where we met up with Phil's family friend, Paul Pelletier. That night, we got a good night's sleep as we were getting ready for our main reason for the trip, the start of the bike ride across the United States!

Today's lesson: If you have a job to do, learn how to do it right and then do it to the best of your ability.

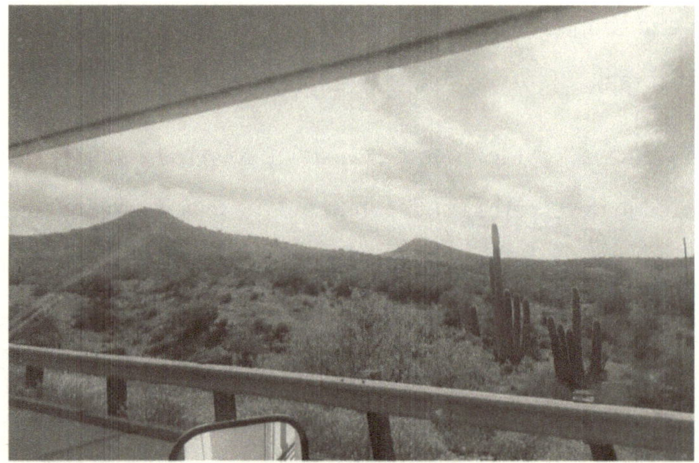

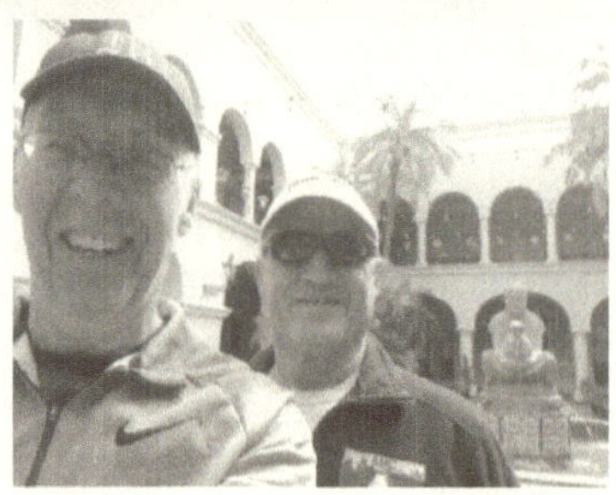

April 17, 2022-Day 9

Day 9 of our trip, Day 1 of our Bike Trip: Happy Easter! This was the day we had been waiting for – the start of our bike ride! We started the day by watching my brother, Fr. David's virtual live mass, celebrating Easter. He did a great job with a beautiful Easter message of new life and new beginnings. We then drove to the Ocean Beach bike path in San Diego, where we placed our bikes into the Pacific Ocean and started our bike trek!

I had the first 25 miles, riding through parts of San Diego, following a GPS map on our phone that was mounted on our bikes. There were times when I did get off the trail and was momentarily lost. However, because of the GPS-guided map, I was able to quickly recover and head back onto the right path. The bike trail quickly left the city limits and headed into the hills of San Diego. I rode through Mission Trail Park, into the towns of Lakeside and Alpine and then across these incredible mountains. The ride was beautiful, going through bike and hiking trails in the hills. Parts of the trail were very hilly, but I did not seem to get tired. There seemed to be a large increase in energy as we started riding our bikes for the first time in a week. It was a great start to a long trip, one that we had been preparing for a long time! It was finally here!

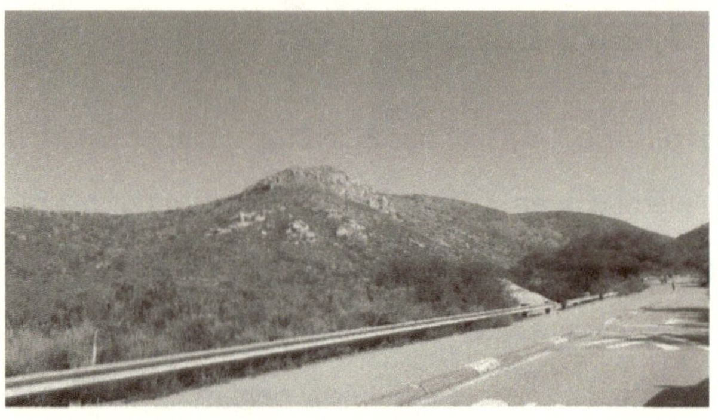

I relayed with Phil in the mountains outside of the City where we made our first switch. Our plan was to have one person ride the bike for 25 miles or so while the other person drove the RV. Then we would switch roles, allowing the bike rider to get a period of rest by driving the RV before repeating the process. We would end up with two sets of 25 miles each (a total of 50 miles each per day), making the total daily ride 100 miles as a Team. The mountains were high, but we kept working at it until we reached the summit at over 4000 feet!

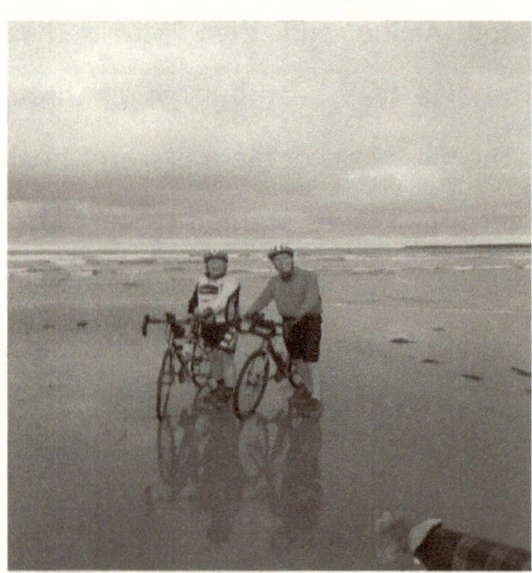

The views of the mountain ranges were spectacular! We descended on the other side of the mountains on our bikes, passing very close to the Mexican border in Jacumba and Calexico, California. We proceeded to a campground in El Centro, California, where we stayed the night, filling up the camper with gas at $5.69 a gallon. It was a long but productive day.

Total miles traveled on bike: 110 miles.

Today's Lesson: All of us will face challenging mountains at some point in our lives. Work hard and be persistent, and you will be successful at reaching the other side someday.

April 18, 2022 – Day 2 of the Bike Ride

We woke up early in the southernmost tip of California. Our original plan was to follow the northern route through more mountains. However, we reviewed the latest update of the maps from our Adventure Cycle resources stating that this particular route had been found to be more dangerous, with many narrow, curvy roads and much truck traffic. So at the last minute, we decided to take an alternate route, going into the most southern part of California and heading north of Yuma, Arizona.

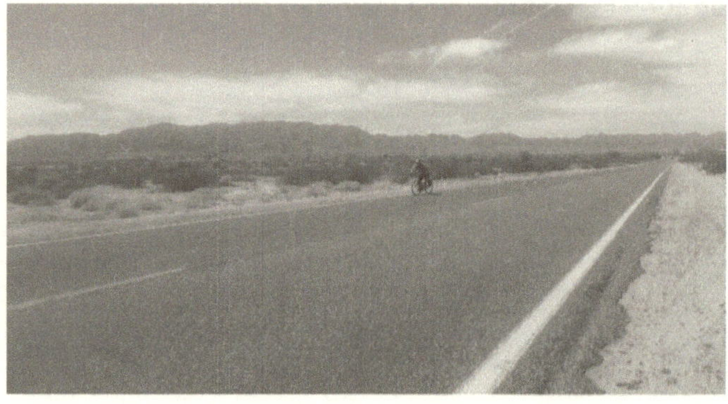

It turned out to be a good decision. The roads were very flat (few hills) and had very little vehicle traffic. However, there were two problems with this decision. First, the roads were somewhat rough in some areas. Second, it was a very hot day to ride the bike, with the temperature reaching 99 degrees most of the afternoon! Even though the roads were not hilly, the temperature was draining!

We kept up our hydration by drinking as much water and Gatorade as we could. The scenery was incredible, with many mountain ranges in the background and mainly desert as far as you could see! Despite the heat and the dry land, we were surprised to see many beautiful farms that grew a variety of vegetables such as lettuce, onions, corn, barley and many other vegetables. Each farm had its own man-made irrigation system of canals, rivers, and water irrigation equipment. The farms were huge, expanding as far as the eye could see! It was beautiful!

That night, we stayed at a campground in Welton, Arizona, taking advantage of their pool. We had a nice meal at a local restaurant and called it an early night, exhausted from the bike ride in the extreme heat.

Total miles traveled on bike: 95 miles.

Today's Lesson: Sometimes, we have to make changes in our plans in life, especially if danger is involved. Many times, these changes can work out for the best. It's okay to take safe risks in life.

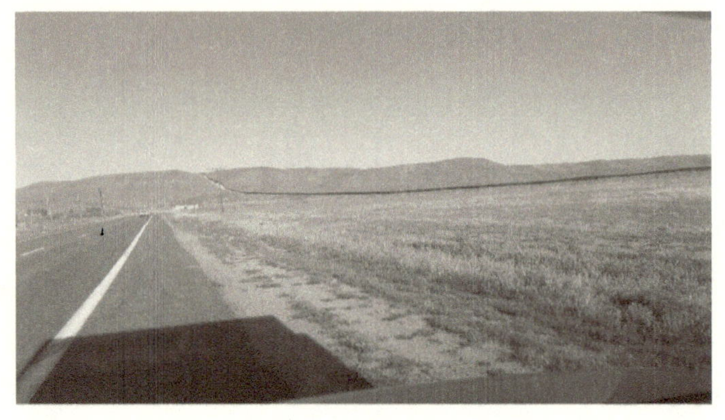

April 19, 2022 – Day 3 of the Bike Ride

After a good night's sleep, we started our ride from the spot where we had left off the day before. I was the first to ride. We left at 5:45 am, very early, to beat the expected heat.

After leaving the town of Tacna, Arizona, I was quickly in the desert area, with the large baron mountains in the background. Even though the landscape was very dry, there was a special beauty to it. There were no cars on this road. I was the only one in this large open area as the sun was rising. It was beautiful. I found myself praying in a way I had never before, thanking God for good health to enjoy this amazing beauty.

The terrain was very flat, so the biking was very fast. (Phil averaged nearly 18 miles an hour, while I averaged 17 miles an hour that day). We each completed 50 miles today in 6.5 hours. By 1:30 pm, we had completed our day, which was a good plan as the temperature had climbed to 99 degrees again today.

As I finished the first leg of my ride, the camper had been parked approximately 200 feet from a railroad track in the middle of the desert. Suddenly, a long, racing freight train came by with cars approximately 2 miles long! The thought immediately came to me about my Dad, who had worked on the railroad all his life (as did my brother, Paul, and my grandfather), and how Dad would have loved to see the site of this long train! He was always so proud of his work on the railroad!

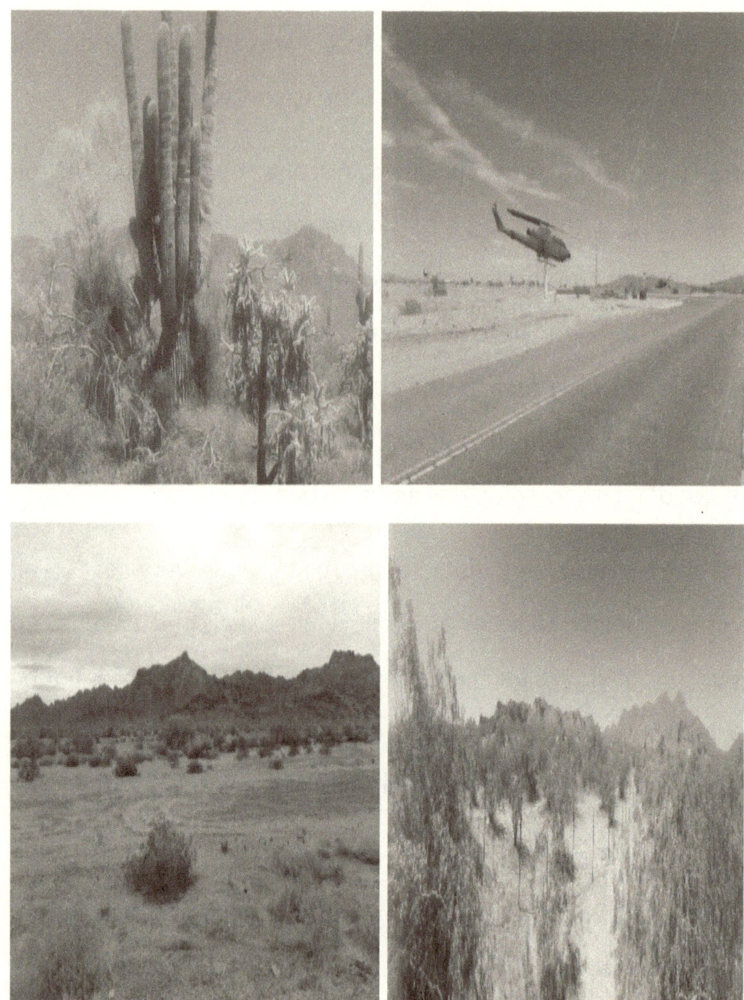

We ended the day in Buckeye, Arizona. We arrived at our campground, took a quick swim in the pool, went shopping for food supplies, ate at a Cracker Barrel restaurant, did laundry, played pool, and settled for the night. Overall, a hot day but a productive day.

Total miles traveled on bike: 100 miles.

Today's Lesson: Take time to appreciate the beauty of this wonderful country. Thank God each day for the gift of health and life.

April 20, 2022 – Day 4 of the Bike Ride

We had another early start out of Buckeye, Arizona. The weather was cool in the morning but warmed to 87 degrees by noon.

Phil started the first leg and did his 25 miles in 1.5 hours. His ride took him through many urban towns outside of Phoenix. He ended up on a bike trail, where we switched riders. Rushing to get started, I forgot to put on my helmet and ended up with my baseball cap instead. It wasn't until 2 miles into the ride that I realized about the forgotten helmet. By then, Phil had already taken off with the camper. I cautiously rode for 38 miles without my helmet, not riding very fast (in fact, my slowest pace yet).

Fortunately, the ride was mostly on a bike path, circulating around Phoenix through Peoria, Mesa, Scottsdale, and finally into Tempe. Riding through the urban areas was eye-opening, with so many homeless people tented on the side of the trail and in the underpasses of highways. In fact, I was riding through a darkened underpass when suddenly, a homeless man leaning against the wall passed out, with his legs sticking out into the trail. At the last second, I saw his white sneakers and turned the bike wheel to the left, missing his foot by less than 6 inches! I continued riding cautiously, finally arriving at Ocean Beach Park in Tempe, Arizona (a beautiful city).

We continued out of the city and into the uphill plateaus of Arizona (one of the prettiest areas so far on our trip), passing through the towns of Sunflower and Jakes Corner. The mountains were amazing as we continued through Tonto National Monument. The biking was a combination of uphills and downhills, expanding across a large mountain range with many tall cacti.

After we had done over 110 miles total for the day, we decided to call it a day and proceeded with the camper to the next available campground, which was not to be found. We ended up staying at a small hotel in Punkin Center, Arizona. After a hot shower and a good meal at the local diner, we ended our day.

Total miles traveled on bike: 113 miles

Today's Lesson #1: Always double-check to ensure you have your safety gear before taking a trip. (Don't forget your helmet)

Today's Lesson #2: You will see some homeless people in your life. Understand that they are not bad people but that many of them have some history of hardship. Instead of offering them money (which they may use for alcohol and drugs), instead, offer them food or water. They are all part of God's creation.

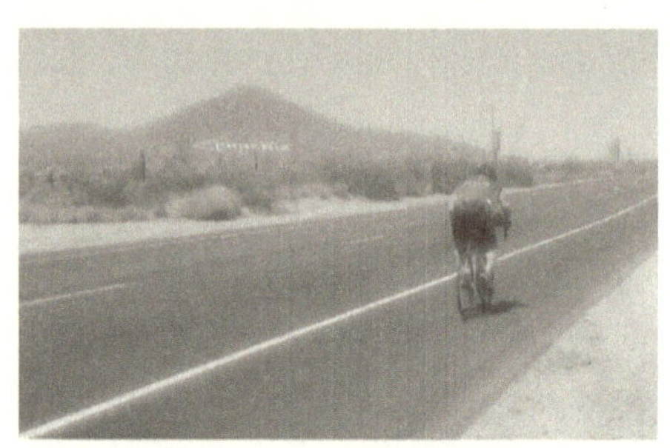

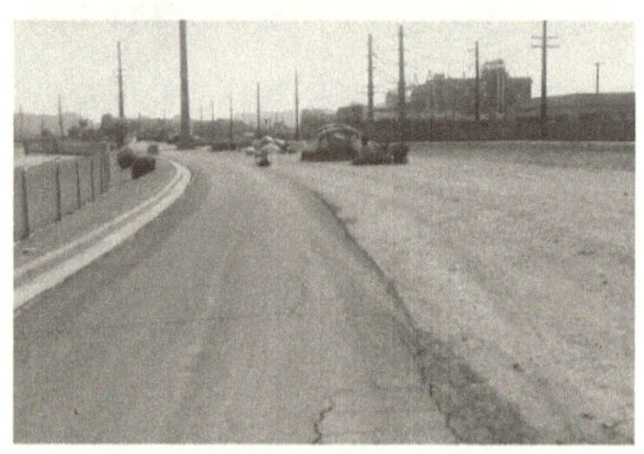

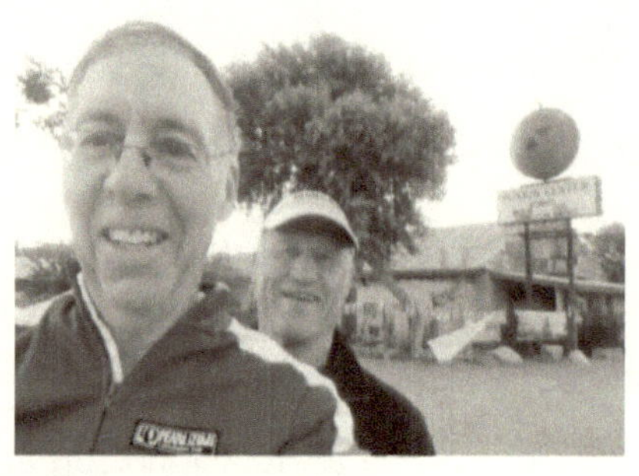

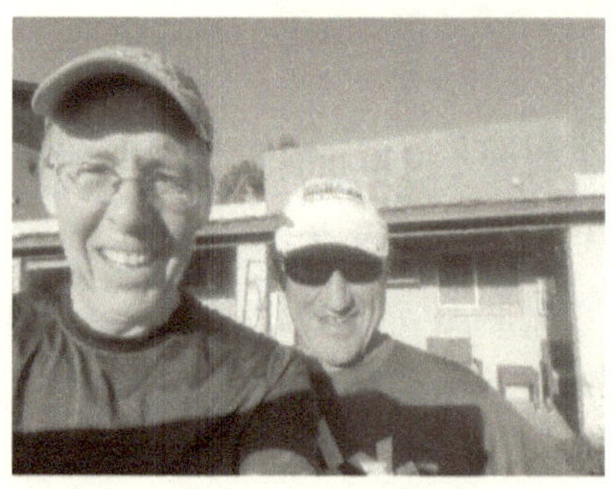

April 21, 2022 – Day 5 of the Bike Ride

Another early start for us. We started biking around 6 am as the sun was just beginning to light up the sky. I did the first leg of the day. It was one of the most beautiful rides so far! I rode into this beautiful valley called Tonto's Basin which contained a small lake surrounded by huge mountains. Many fishing boats passed by on their way to the lake. There were only slight hills with many downhills, which made for an easy ride. I had to stop multiple times to take panoramic pictures of the scenery. What beauty God has created, I told myself as I rode the 25 miles.

I continued riding through the area until reaching the town of Roosevelt. Phil was waiting for me there to change positions. He started his portion of the ride only to meet a very large mountain climb of over 2000 feet in less than 3 miles. As I passed him with the camper noticing that this was going to be an incredible bike climb, I called him on the phone and asked if he wanted me to pick him up and have him ride up the hill in the camper. He said, "No, I want to challenge myself and see if I can do it." Well, he did it without stopping!

Once he had reached the top, he had an easy 10-mile downhill ending in Globe, Arizona. There, we switched riders again and headed out of town on Route 70. We continued for an additional 50 miles through the Apache territory of southeast Arizona with a continued desert landscape surrounded by huge mountains.

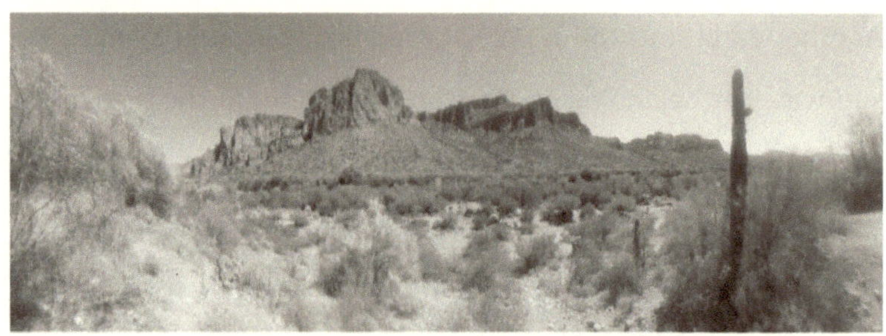

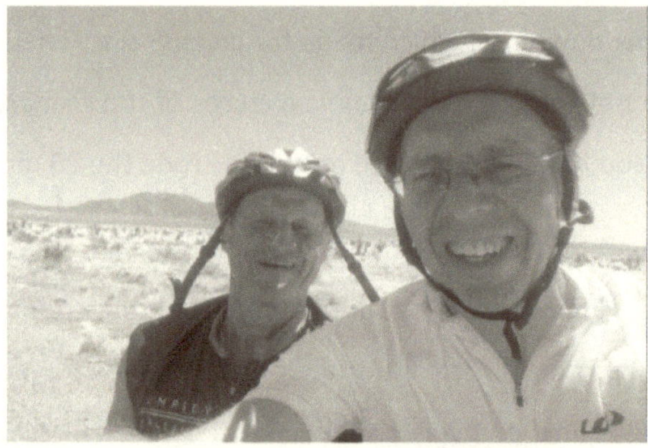

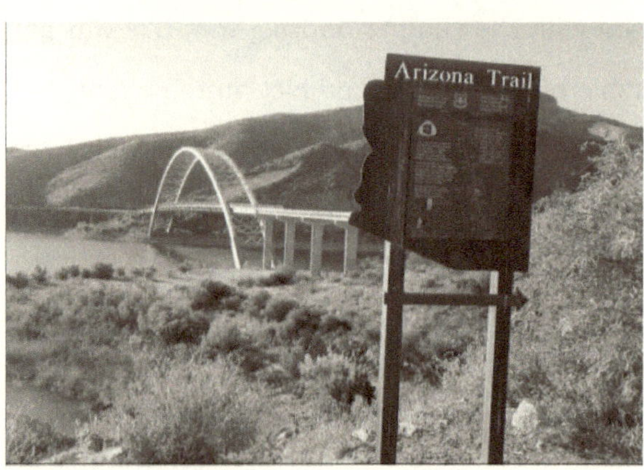

We passed through the small towns of Peridot and Geronimo. These were important towns in the past, but time had taken traffic away from these areas and replaced them with interstate travel systems many miles away. The small amount of traffic was fast, and the road shoulders were narrow on this road. We took our time and rode safely to our campground in Thatcher, Arizona.

Total miles traveled on bike: 100 miles.

Today's Lesson: In life, we will all face large uphills that will challenge us. Stay strong during those times, and you will reach the summit and enjoy the wonderful rewards.

April 22, 2022 – Day 6 of the Bike Ride

When I woke up this morning, I had a strong feeling that today was going to be different... and it was. Phil started the first bike phase out of Thatcher, Arizona, and I drove ahead of him with the camper. It was a sunny but cool start to the day. The first part of the ride was through large prairie fields surrounded by huge mountains. I stopped a few times on the way to take pictures of the scenery. The roads we biked on today were ideal, with wide shoulders and much less traffic. We switched riders in Duncan, Arizona, the last town before crossing into New Mexico.

My first segment for biking was almost ideal conditions with a slight breeze on my right side. The land was mostly desert as I rode on Route 70 through Franklin and ended near Lordsburg, New Mexico. By the time my second segment came along, the wind had really picked up. By then, we were off Route 70 and onto Route 90, heading towards The Gila Highlands of New Mexico. The road looked very flat, but when I looked at my speedometer, I noted that I was going very slowly, despite a strong tailwind. Glancing at the elevation traveled, I could see that even though it looked flat, there was actually a significant increase in the elevation! As I kept on riding, the hills really started to get steeper.

At that point, I was ready to call Phil to pick me up with the camper. Then I asked for God's help. I said, "God, I don't think I can make this alone. You have to help me." Suddenly, a tailwind picked up, helping to push me up the hill. If the road curved a certain way, the tailwind would shift in the same direction I was heading. As the hills got steeper, the wind got stronger to help me. This continued for miles. (Total elevation biked that day was nearly 3000 feet).

As I got closer to one of the summits and was racing downhill, the wind suddenly shifted and was now directly to my left side, pushing the total bike nearly off the road to the right. About halfway down this large hill, I suddenly saw a large gray-colored snake (serpent) over 3 feet long directly in my bike track! I swerved to the left, trying to avoid hitting the snake. As I got closer to the bottom of the hill, the wind suddenly changed direction again, back to a tailwind, helping me go up the challenging hills. The wind was so soothing. It seemed that every time I asked God to help me with the uphill, the wind would get stronger to help me. At times, the wind pushed me up the hill without me even pedaling! It was the closest that I have ever been in my life to actually touching God. I did not understand this event's reasoning, but I wanted to find out. (Like Moses and the burning bush, or the theme of the movie "Field of Dreams"). I continued on my path, passing my planned stop for many miles, trying to find out what God was telling me. Was this the reason for the bike trip? Or was there something else he wanted me to know? I still did not have the answer despite now arriving at our night destination of Silver City, New Mexico. It was an incredible experience!

Total mileage today: 117 miles and 3020 feet of elevation.

Today's Lesson: God has many ways of communicating with you directly. Be open to His signs.

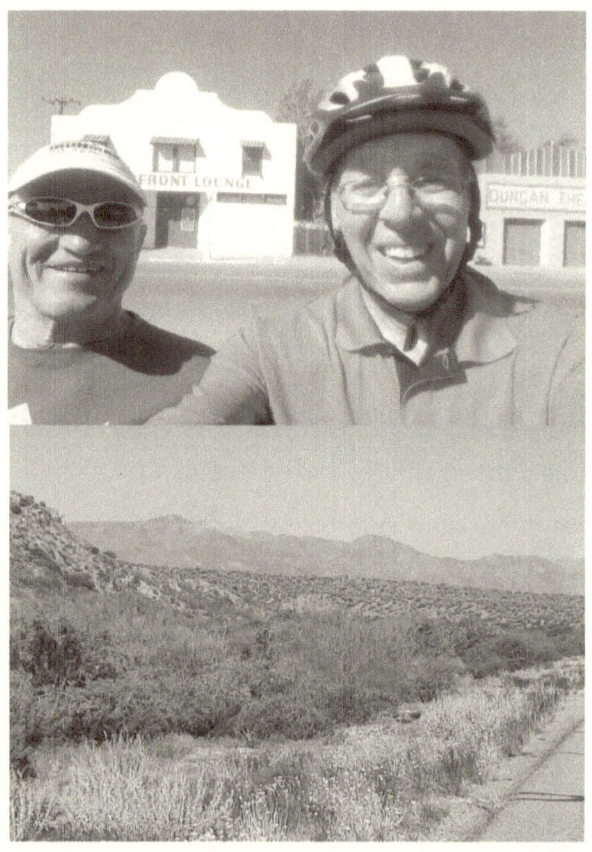

April 23, 2022 – Day 7 of the Bike Ride

We are now one week into our bike ride. Our spirits and bodies are doing well. (It is amazing how much work the body can do!) Today was a cold start (45 degrees) and a difficult first leg for both of us. We were riding in the Gila National Forest, where the lady in charge of the campground stated some bikers were staying at their campground while training for the Tour de France. That is when we knew we would be in for challenging hill work!

After starting on today's ride, we understood what she meant. There were many uphill mountains in our path. (I accented 2300 feet in the first 25 miles.), reaching a height of over 7000 feet. Fortunately, the roads were in good shape, and the traffic was very light. At one point, there were over ten deer that passed in front of me on the road. They were mainly fawns with three adult deer. They saw me and quickly ran into the woods. These were the first true wildlife seen on my travels so far. They were beautiful!

My second leg was much better, mainly on flat prairies surrounded by high mountains, through the towns of Kingston, Hillsboro, by Caballo Lake, and ending in the town of Cappello. Phil switched with me at that point and rode through Arrey, Derry Hatch and Rincon, New Mexico.

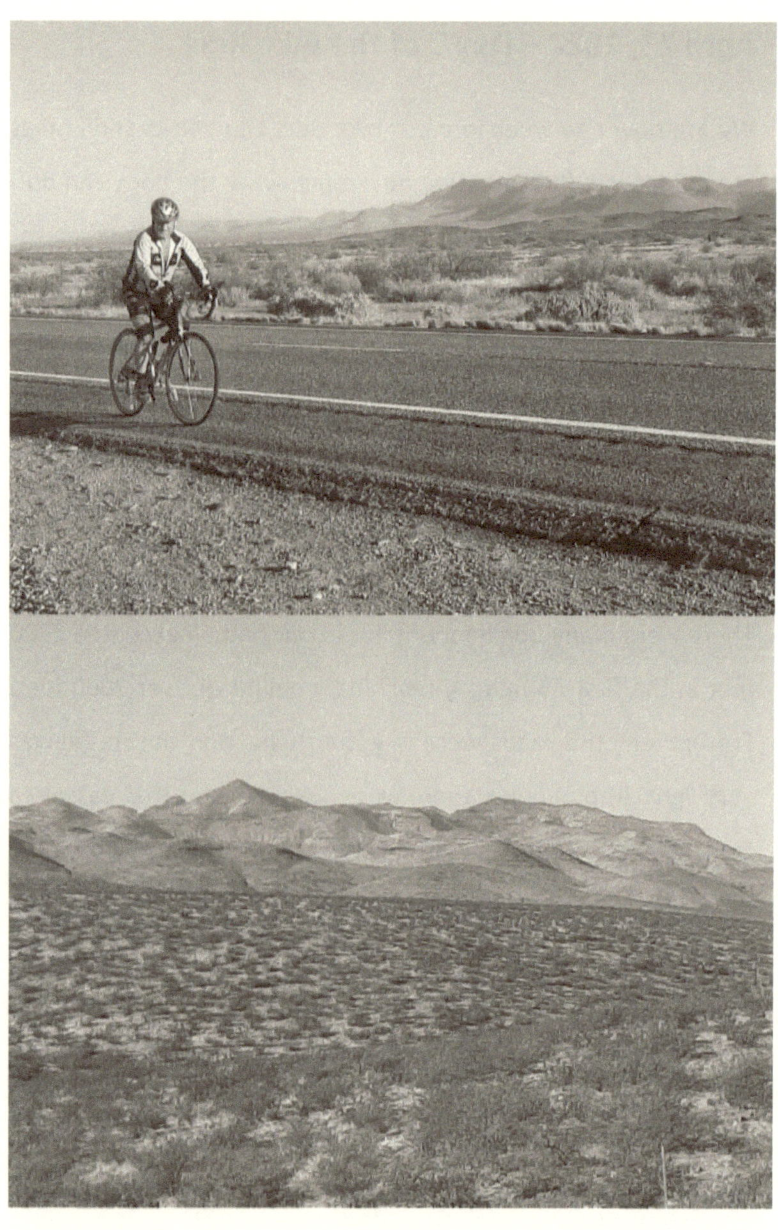

During my rest stop, I received a call from a person who was a
potential kidney donor for a friend of mine in Florida. (I had

shared my number with my friend to see if he had any questions about life after an organ donation since I had donated one of my kidneys to my brother in 2013). When I told him I was presently biking across the country, it didn't take long to answer many of his questions. He was very thankful and reassured about his physical abilities after the donation. After we had each completed our 50 miles that day, we each added another 10 miles of biking so that we would end in Las Cruces, New Mexico. We found a KOA campground, had dinner at a local Cracker Barrel Restaurant and called it a day. It had been a challenging day of biking.

Total miles traveled on bike: 120 miles.

Today's Lesson #1: The human body is an incredible machine. Please take good care of it with proper diet and exercise.

Today's Lesson #2: The wildlife is so precious. Make sure you do everything possible to protect it.

April 24, 2022 – Day 8 of the Bike Trip

We left Las Cruces, New Mexico, by 6 am. It was a perfect day to bike with the warm temperature, tailwind, and flat landscape. I had the second leg of the bike ride, which started north of El Paso, Texas. We passed many farms with well-groomed trees of pecan for many miles. I was enjoying the scenery and ride so much that I was not paying attention to the route GPS and went past the turnoff by over one mile.

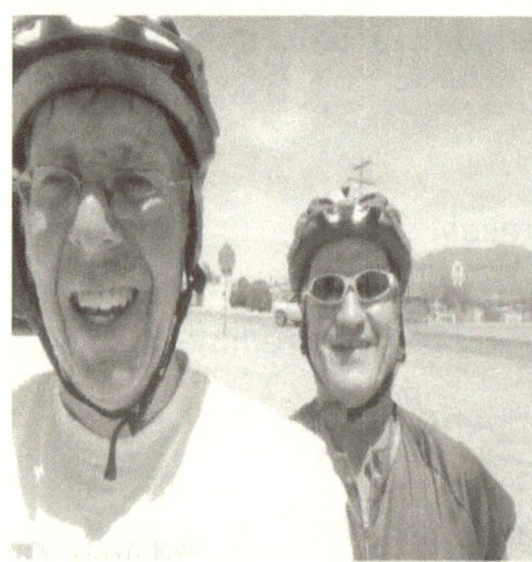
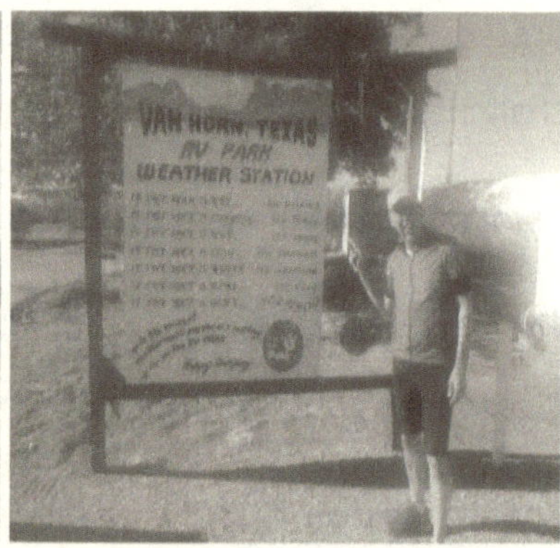

Once I realized the mistake, I had to retrace the route, losing time and energy. The turnoff brought me to a great bike path, which I followed for several miles, ending just north of El Paso, Texas. Phil was waiting for me there with the camper. We drove the camper through the busy downtown area of El Paso, where we continued our bike ride outside the city. El Paso looked like a very nice city which I hope to visit in more detail in the future.

Once we were out of the city, the traffic was very light, and the conditions were perfect. We did not seem to get tired. We rode on back roads, following the Rio Grande River on the border of Mexico. We rode over 135 miles, passing many small towns such as Tornillo, Fort Hancock and Sierra Blanca, ending in Van Horn, Texas, where we switched to Central Time. After a good meal at a local restaurant, we called it a very productive day.

Total miles traveled on bike: 135 miles.

Today's Lesson: It is important to pay close attention to direction details. Always plan and know where you are traveling.

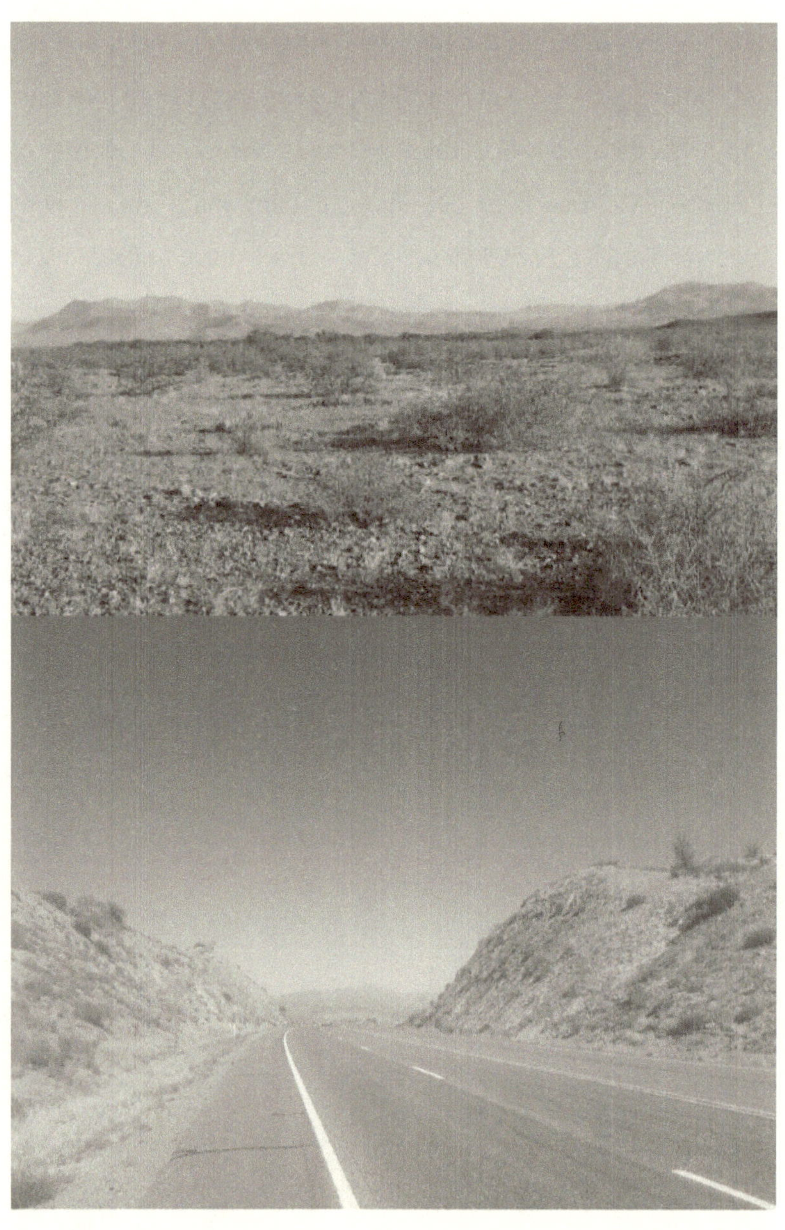

April 25, 2022 - Day 9 of the Bike Trip

We started the day at sunrise in Van Horn, Texas. I had the first leg of 25 miles. It was a cool morning at 55 degrees. The first leg went very well; flat terrain, good road, no traffic, and no major towns.

However, a headwind soon picked up. We went through mostly desert land, crossing through only one small town of Valentine. Phil had the second leg of the ride, which was mostly a slight uphill with a much stiffer wind. By the time I did my second leg, the wind was now blowing at 25 to 30 mph, almost at a direct headwind and uphill for more than 18 of the next 25 miles! The ride was very tough, lasting over 2 hours. I struggled to reach Marfa, Texas, a very small but artistic town with great signage and colorful storefronts. As I passed through the town, a group of people gathered to listen to live music in one of the outdoor cafés. My trek continued past Marfa, where Phil was waiting for me to do the last leg of the day. My body was tired, and I needed rest. Therefore, the rest of the day was filled with rest, hydration and a good warm meal. We ended the day in a campground in Alpine, Texas, one of the most exhausting days of our ride so far.

Total miles traveled on bike: 95 miles.

Today's Lesson: The body is an incredible machine. However, you must listen to your body when it is tired and make sure to get the proper rest, hydration and nutritious food.

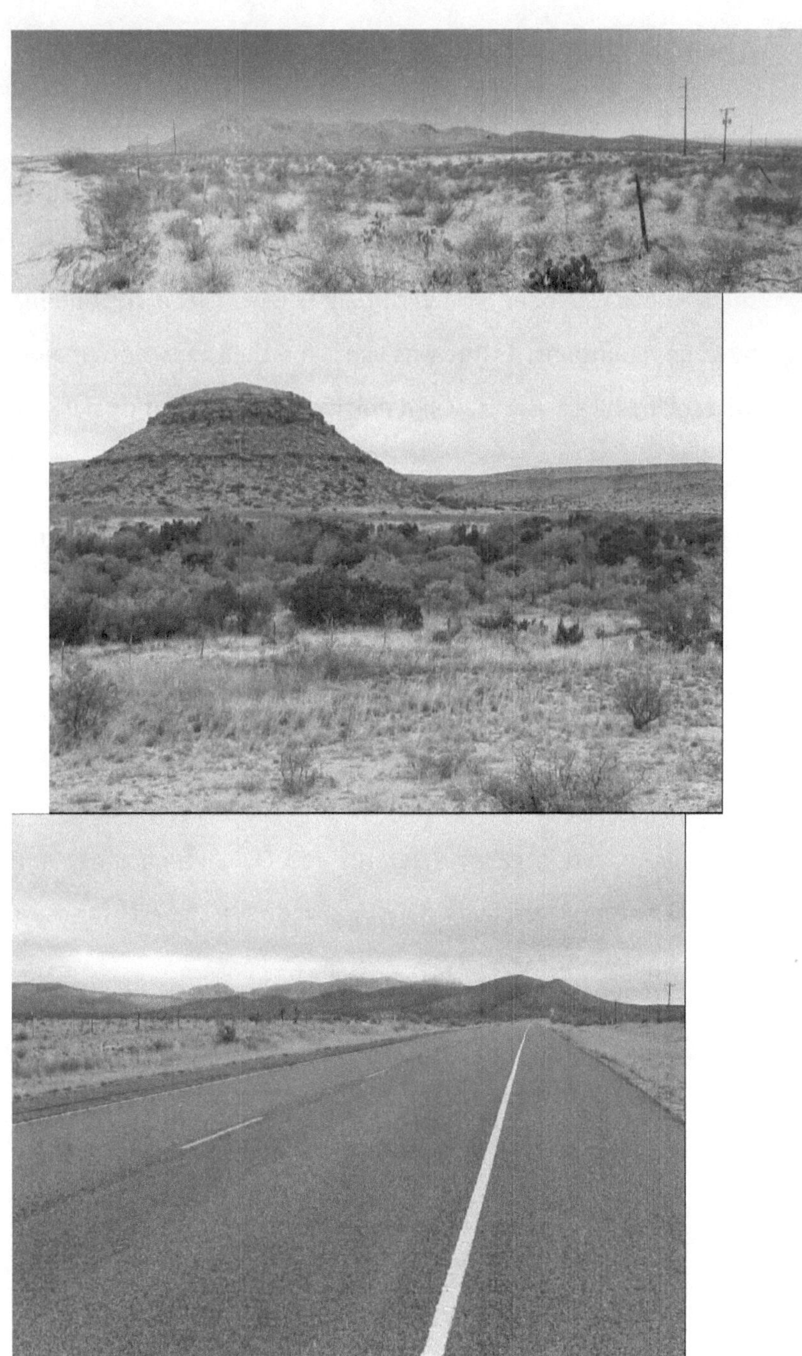

April 26, 2022 – Day 10

We started in Alpine, Texas, early in the morning. It was another cool morning at 55 degrees, and we had an 8 mph headwind all day! It was very tough biking despite very few hills. However, the scenery was beautiful, with mainly desert land surrounded by large mountains. Traffic was light, and the roads were mainly mild rolling hills as we traveled north of Big Bend National Park.

On my first leg of the ride, the only town we passed was Marathon, with a population of about 400 people. On my second leg, I met up with a biker who was also doing the same Southern Tier bike route that we were following. He started telling me his story – a seven-year survivor of stage 4 cancer. His wife, who was driving the support camper, also had cancer and was still undergoing treatment. Together, they started a non-profit organization called "Get Up and Live." Their story and positive energy were incredibly inspiring! We shared stories as we rode together for miles.

Later that evening, we all got together at the campground with other riders in a town called Sanderson, Texas, to share our journey experiences. It was motivating. We felt blessed to meet these inspiring people. We are finding out that everyone who does this bike ride has a unique reason to do this milestone journey. Some reasons we know beforehand, while others we experience on the way. It is a time to evaluate your life: where you've been, where you are presently, and where you're going. It is turning into a true Pilgrimage.

Total miles traveled on bike: 84 miles.

Today's Lesson: Sometimes life gives us challenges (Headwinds, cancer, etc.). However, through hard work, blessings, and positive attitudes, these challenges can be overcome. Stay positive!

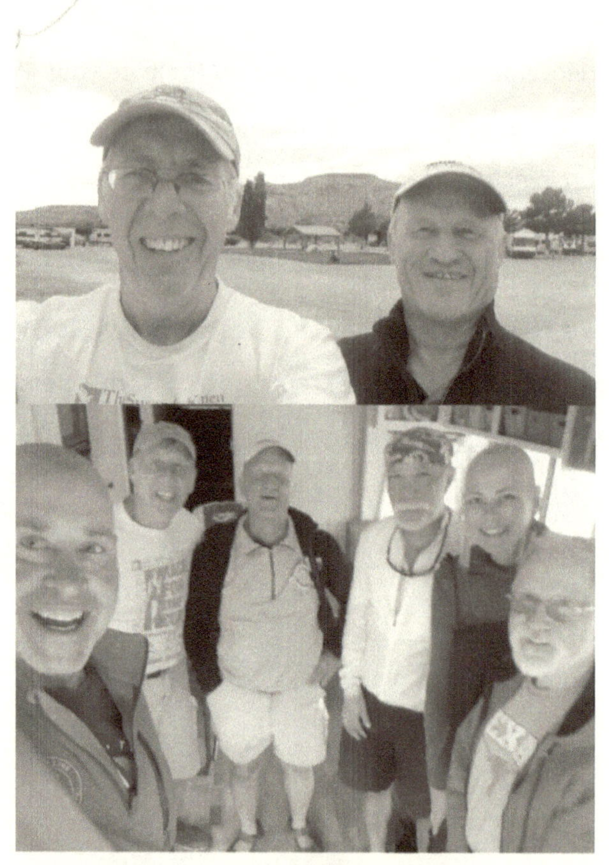

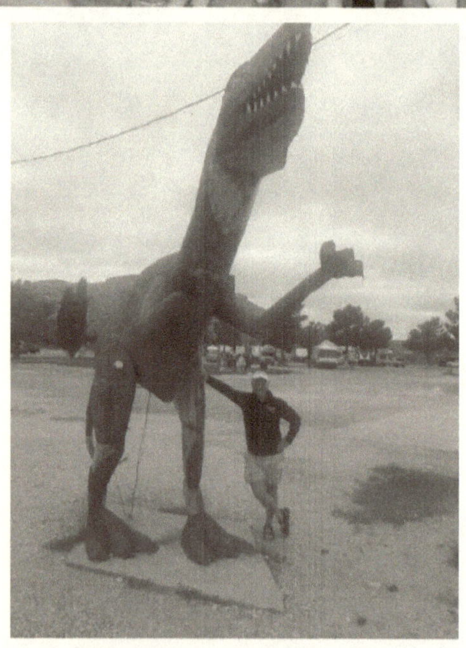

April 27, 2022 – Day 11 of the Bike Ride

Today's ride would bring us through the dry prairies of west Texas, following the Rio Grande River, very close to the Mexican border. There were Border Patrolmen everywhere! I even saw four Mexican-appearing gentlemen on the side of the road in the middle of nowhere, just sitting and waiting for a ride. Being so close to the border through deserted terrain, we saw very little traffic. We had checked the weather forecast the night before and knew it was going to be a challenging day with headwinds of 10 to 20 mph. We were also determined to reach Del Rio, Texas, which was 110 miles away. With that in mind, I had the first leg and took off just as the sun was rising over the mountains. At that time of day, the winds were calm, and the ride was great!

However, as the morning continued, so came the high winds. It was now getting much harder to ride as we started to get physically tired. We knew we needed to switch our plans. So we made two changes. First, we overlapped our switches by having the camper driver start his ride 5 miles before the other person arrived. Second, we shortened our rides to 15 miles per leg instead of the usual 25 miles. This would give us a quicker time to rest and recover between shifts. It worked very well, and we were able to achieve our goal by reaching Del Rio, Texas, by 2:30 pm, after riding through the small towns of Dryden,

Langtry and Comstock. During that ride, there were 89 miles of road that had no services for food, drink, or camping. We were tired but pleased that we had reached our goal distance by arriving at Del Rio!

Total miles traveled on bike: 110 miles.

Today's Lesson: Sometimes when the conditions are not quite right, you have to adjust your plans in order to reach your goal. If you are flexible with your plans, you may be more successful.

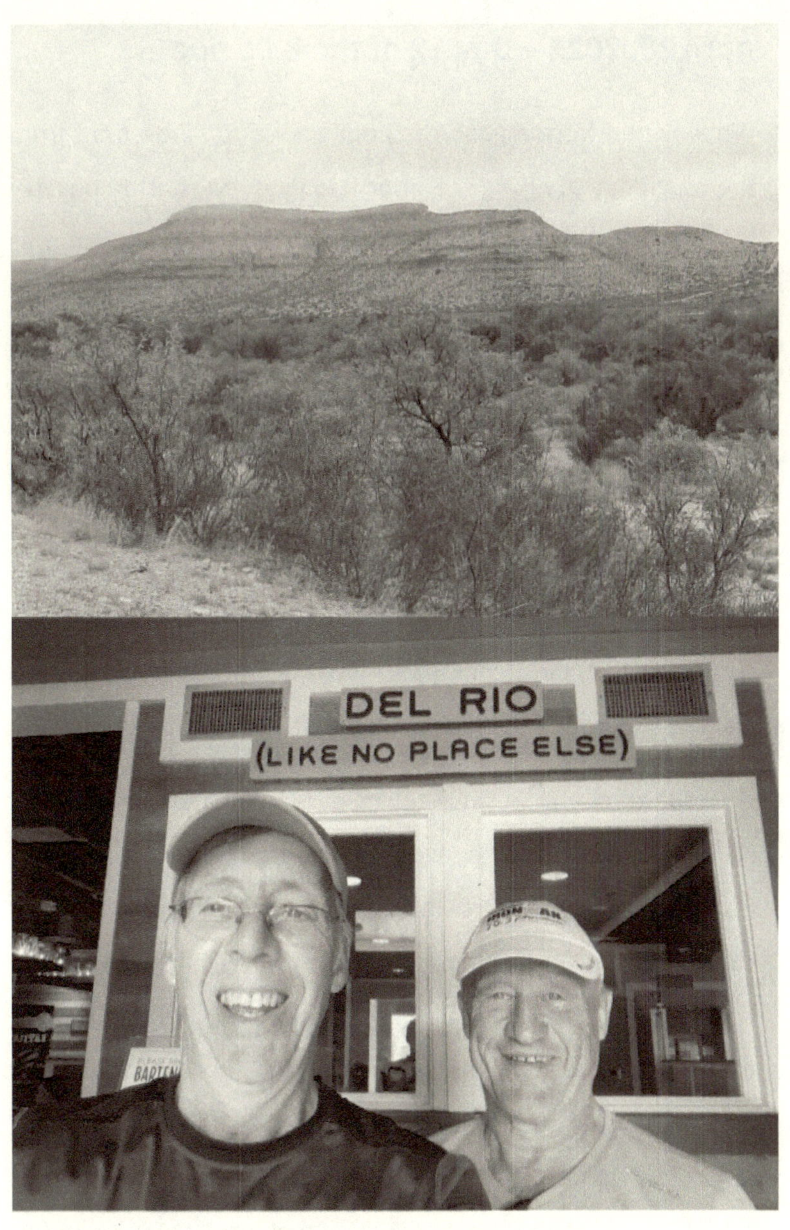

DEL RIO
(LIKE NO PLACE ELSE)

April 28, 2022 – Day 12 of the Bike ride

We woke up from a good rest, our bodies still a bit tired from the tough day of biking the prior two days. We started our day just outside Del Rio, Texas. Phil had the first leg which was through some fast traffic on Route 90. His biking lane was also rough, causing his arms to get numb from the vibration. I had a more pleasant ride on Route 334 out of Bracketville, where the traffic was very light (less than ten cars in 25 miles of riding), and the road was pretty smooth for biking. What was quickly noticeable was that the trees were now taller and greener than we had seen since California. There were also many small cattle ranches with their arched gates identifying their ranch names, just like we used to see on the television show Bonanza!

We rode through the small towns of Montell and Camp Wood. My second leg of the ride was totally different. It was very hilly (over 2300 feet elevation in 25 miles) - including the steepest climb I had experienced on the ride so far! We ended the day in a town called Leaky, Texas, totally exhausted. We had a great meal outside at a friendly restaurant and then had a difficult time finding a campground that offered showers. Someone suggested Garner State Park, about 8 miles down a different road from our route. What a blessing that was! It was beautiful! Our campsite was near a small lake surrounded by majestic mountains and huge trees. We had a pleasant walk near the lake and then sat down to relax and review the day.

Total miles traveled on bike: 95 miles.

Today's Lesson: Sometimes, we are blessed with great beauty and wonderful experiences when we least expect them. Always keep your eyes open for these pleasant surprises.

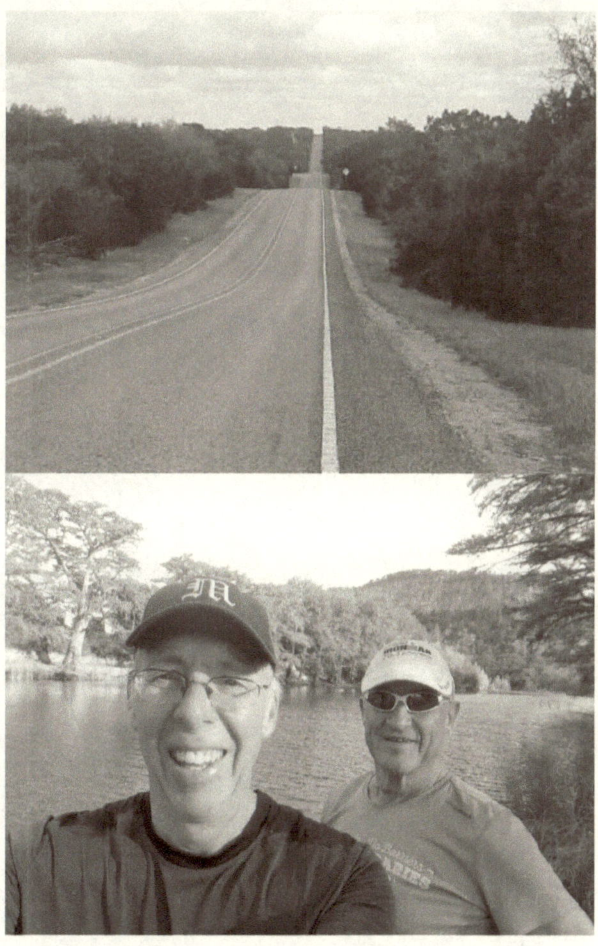

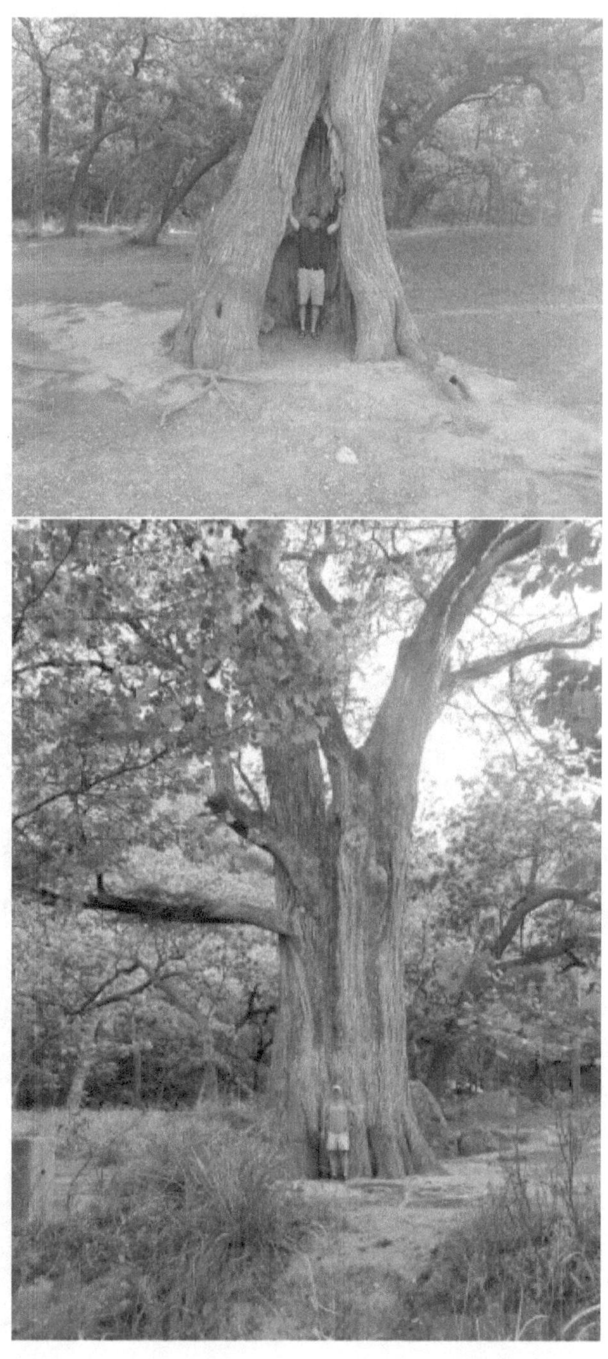

April 29, 2022 – Day 13 of the Bike Ride

We left Leakey, Texas, early in the morning, only to find that the State Park where we were staying had locked gates to get out until 7:30 am. Fortunately, a Park Ranger arrived and let us out at 7 am. We then started our ride out of the town of Leakey. I had the first leg of the bike ride that day. The weather was in the 60s, but there was a mist of rain throughout my first 25 miles. Plus, there were very steep hills just outside of town. The ride was miserable! It took over 2 hours to do the first 25 miles, going over very steep hills to an elevation of 2500 feet. We continued into a town called Kerrville, which has a population of over 22,000 people. The map was confusing, and the internet reception was spotty. Phil had been biking for about 20 miles and was getting tired. We decided to both stop and have lunch. It was one of the few times on the trip that we actually had lunch together as we took a lunch break at a local Subway shop.

When we left, I rode the camper and followed what I thought was the correct trail on the GPS. However, the GPS system was "frozen" and had sent me off course by miles. As I waited for Phil to arrive, he called me and said, "Where are you? I have already gone my 25 miles and do not see the camper." It was then that I realized that I had missed a turnoff and was way off course. So I quickly backtracked to find Phil. By then, he had continued on the back roads of Texas, where there was no traffic. Cows were grazing loosely in the roads and fields! I finally caught up to Phil about 20 miles further than planned. I was very sorry. He was very forgiving and said that it was okay, despite being very late. We continued to bike ride, and each did an extra 10 miles more than planned, ending up in Johnson City, Texas. After a shower at the local campground and a very good Mexican meal, we visited the boyhood home of Lyndon B. Johnson, our 36th President.

Total miles traveled on bike: 120 miles.

Today's Lesson: Good Friends are people who can forgive you, even when you make a mistake. Always do your best to support your friends.

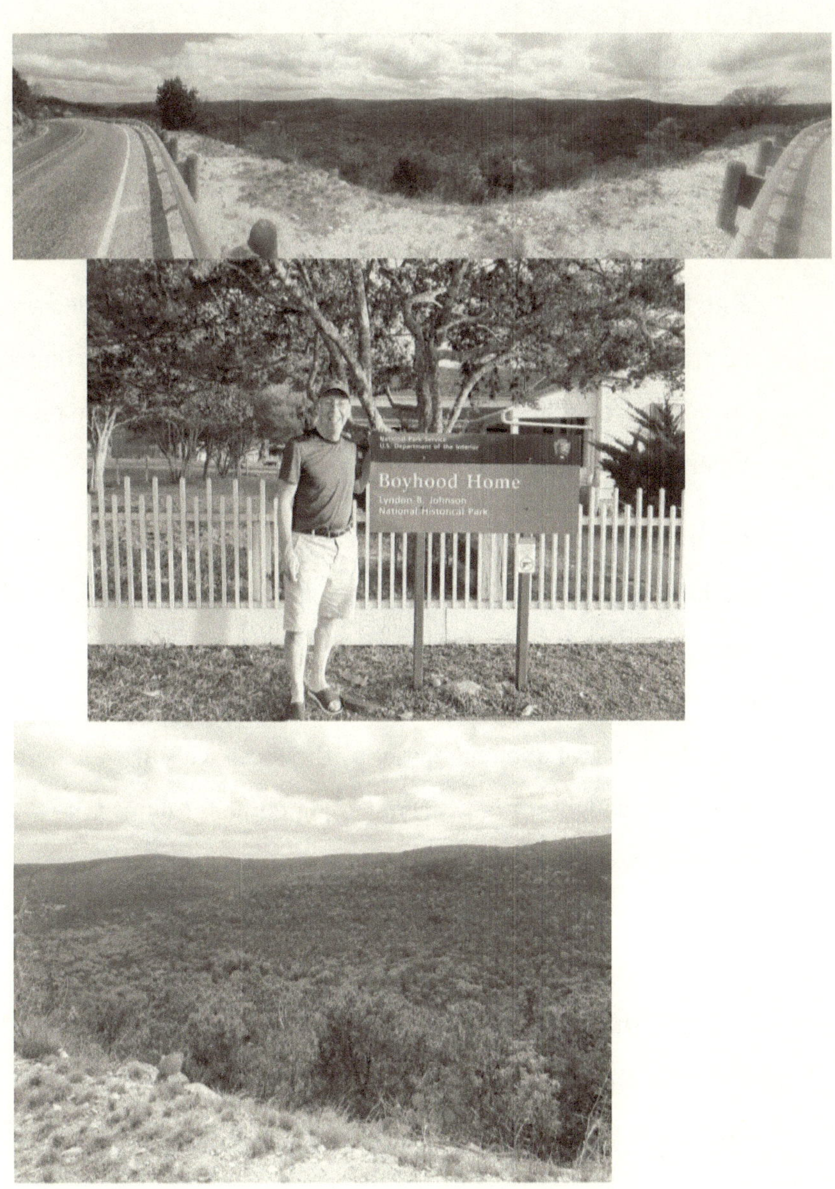
National Park Service
U.S. Department of the Interior
Boyhood Home
Lyndon B. Johnson
National Historical Park

April 30, 2022 – Day 14 of the Bike Ride

Today was a day of rest. After biking for 13 straight days, we decided to give our bodies (and minds) a day off. Although we were not sore in our muscles, our minds were tired from the large focus needed each day for a successful ride. We called an old friend, Robert Dumais, a high school friend from Northern Maine who now lives in the San Antonio area. I had not seen Robert for over 40 years!

We traveled to his beautiful home, where we met his wife, mother-in-law and even one of his daughters and two of his eight grandchildren. They were all very welcoming. We rode with Robert to the downtown area of San Antonio where we visited the Alamo and had dinner by the River Walk. It was there that Phil's daughter-in-law, Natalie, joined us for dinner. It was great to visit everyone and to give our bodies and minds a break! Even though we had not seen each other for decades, our conversations were easy, as if we had seen each other recently. That night, we headed back to Cedar Creek, Texas, where we stayed at a campground for the night. Overall, a good day of rest!

Total miles traveled on bike: 0 miles

Today's Lesson #1: It is okay to take a day off for rest when you have been working hard. Your mind and body will need it!

Today's Lesson #2: Old Friends are a true gift. It is good to connect with them whenever possible. Don't miss an opportunity to visit them.

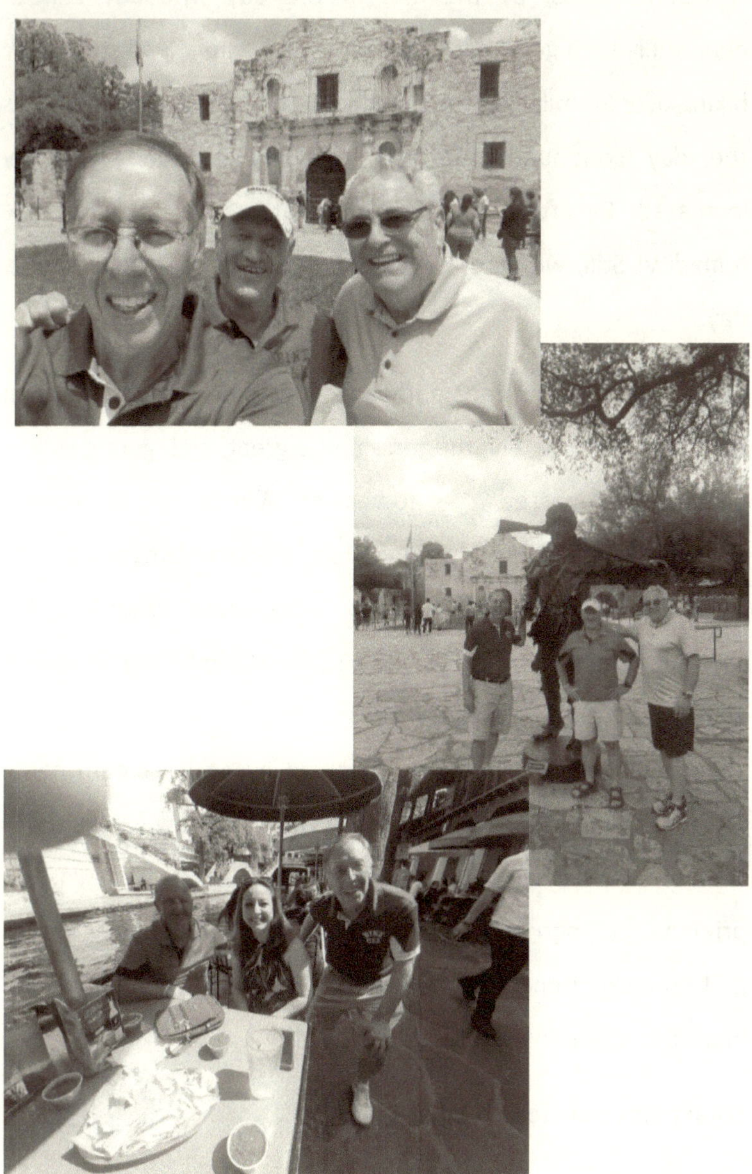

May 1, 2022 - Day 15 of the Bike Ride

We left Cedar Creek, Texas, at sunrise. Our goal was to reach Navasota, Texas, by the end of the day. The day started beautifully with good back roads and rare traffic. Phil started by biking over 20 miles on the quiet roads of Bastrop State Park. As the day continued, the sun got stronger, and humidity increased. By afternoon, the temperature was 90 with 77% humidity! Still, we were determined to reach our goal for the day.

Both of us hydrated constantly and slowed our speed by pacing ourselves. Fortunately, the terrain was great, with gentle rolling hills as we passed the towns of Winchester, LaGrange, Oldenburg, Warrenton, Round Top, Burton, Longpoint, and Independence. We did run into a bike race fundraiser for Multiple Sclerosis on the way. By 3:30 pm, we had reached our goal by arriving in Navasota, Texas. We enjoyed a nice meal at an outside café in Navasota, followed by an ice cream cone. (This was a real treat for us!) There were very few campsites in the area, so we had to travel about 16 miles out of town to a primitive campground with one old outdoor shower. It was quite the experience! We called it an early night, trying to sleep in a warm camper without electricity.

Total miles traveled on bike: 115 miles.

Today's Lesson: Conditions in life are not always ideal. Sometimes, if you want to reach your goals, you have to modify your speed and increase your patience while continuing to pace yourself. It is then that you will be successful.

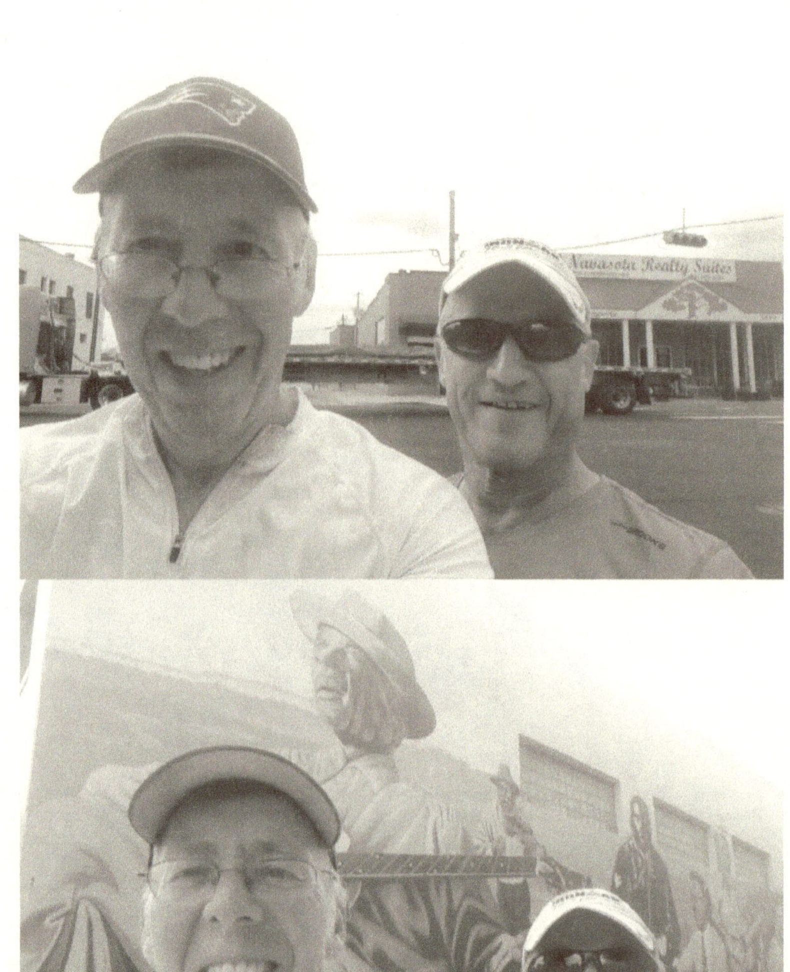

May 2, 2022 - Day 16 of the Bike Trip

We found out the reason we did not see our campground owners last night when we checked in was because they were involved in a local charity bicycle race to raise money for the Multiple Sclerosis Foundation. Once we heard that they were helping a good cause, it was difficult to be upset about our difficulty in getting settled into the campground last night.

After having a poor night's sleep, we left our basic campground by sunrise and headed for the downtown area of Navasota to start the first leg of today's bike ride. The weather conditions started ideal, with low wind and the temperature in the low 70s. The road started with fast traffic on Route 90, but we quickly took the side road off Route 149, which had very little traffic and few hills. Road conditions for most of the day were almost ideal, and we made a very good time. However, the temperature got much warmer, topping off at 90 degrees.

Fortunately, the trees on the side of the road were now much taller and greener in this part of the state, causing more shade and sheltering us from the sun and the winds. Overall, despite a tough start at our old campground, it was a good day. We rode through the towns of Anderson, New Waverly, Coldspring, Shepherd, and Kountze and ended up in Silsbee, Texas, for the night. We took the camper and drove south to Lumberton for dinner and to pick up a few things at the supermarket. We had a cold swim at the campground pool and settled in for the night.

Total miles traveled on bike: 120 miles.

Today's Lesson: It is important to support non-profit organizations and to find a charity that you are passionate about supporting. It may not help you financially, but you will feel warmth in your heart that will have true meaning to you. Make sure to give part of yourself to others without expecting something in return.

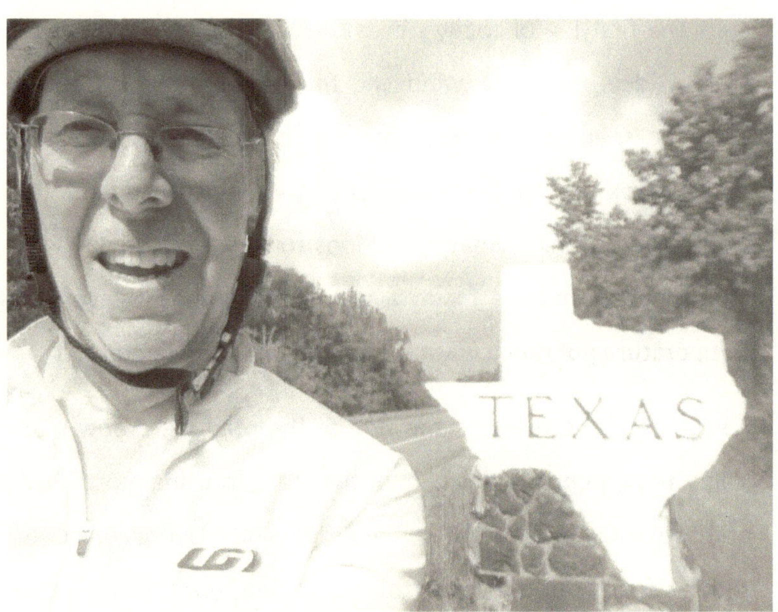

May 3, 2022 – Day 17 of the Bike Ride

We had a good start out of Silsbee, Texas, leaving at sunrise around 6:45. Both of us had great rides, quickly accumulating 50 miles in less than 3.5 hours. During that time, we did cross the border from Texas into Louisiana!

As Phil was halfway through his second leg of the day, it started to rain – at first a gentle rain, then more steady rain. (It was the first real rain we had seen so far on our bike trip.) I pulled up next to him in the camper and offered to come in and dry up with new clothes. "No. I think the rain is slowing down. I will keep on going," said Phil. "Are you sure, Phil? The forecast is giving rain for the next 2 hours," said I. "No," he replied. "I will keep on going." So he did.

It wasn't more than 15 minutes later when the sky opened up with very heavy rain. By the time I could catch up to him, he had taken refuge in a Porta potti at a construction site on the side of the road. He called me and let me know his location. When I arrived, he came into the camper dripping wet, along with his bike. He quickly changed into warm clothes.

We waited for about 2 hours in the camper, playing cards and waiting for the sun to come out. As predicted, the sun came out, and the rest of the day was sunny with hot, humid weather. We completed the ride that day, passing through the towns of

Buna, Kirbyville, Merryville, DeRidder and Oberin, ending up in Mamou, Louisiana. Our campsite was in Eunice, Louisiana, in the middle of Cajun Country. We had a Cajun meal of catfish that night and returned to a nice campground for the night.

Total miles traveled on bike: 125 miles.

Today's Lesson: It's okay to be stubborn at times, as long as it is for a positive reason — and not to be done for just being different and falsely bold. Always use your "stubbornness" in a positive way.

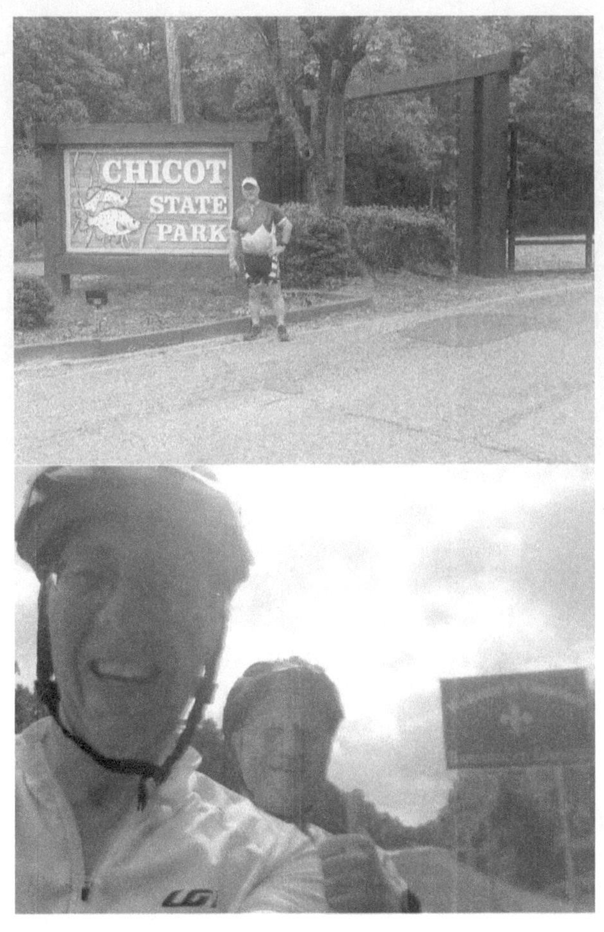

CHICOT
STATE
PARK

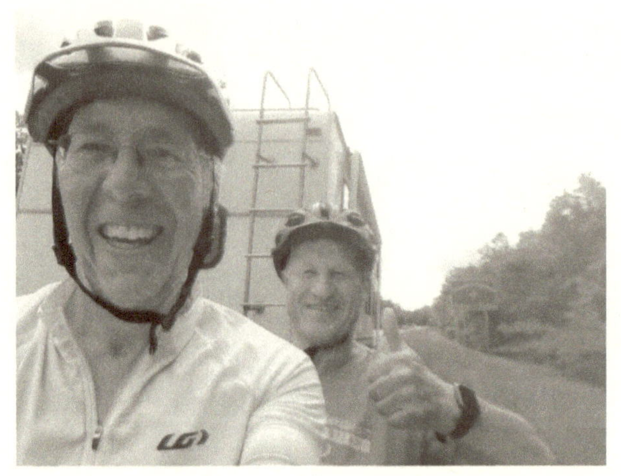

May 4, 2022 – Day 18

Today was one of the most memorable days of the trip. We started the bike ride early in the morning, starting in downtown Mamou, Louisiana – the heart of Cajun country and part of our Acadian heritage. The small town was deserted at that time of day, but the buildings were like something out of a movie. The nightclubs that ring out Zydeco music were everywhere, including the famous "Fred's Place."

The bike route continued by many flooded rice fields and other agricultural farms. It was interesting to see how they used their irrigation systems to nurture their fields, similar to the original Acadians of Port Royal, Nova Scotia. We continued our ride to the small town of Ville Patte, Louisiana, where we stopped at a cemetery to see if we could find similar Acadian family names from our St. John Valley roots. We were able to find names such as Picard, Hebert and Dupre, but no Raymond's, Roy's, Dufour's, or Albert's.

As we biked through town, the cultural resemblance to the St. John Valley was amazing! The architecture of the homes and businesses, the street landscape, the small business signs, and the Churches all reminded us of our Family home in northern Maine. It was amazing that two totally different areas of the country with similar Acadian roots in the 1700s could look so much alike! It was very comforting.

We biked on the flat back roads of Cajun country most of the day, passing through towns such as St. Landry, Bunkie, Cottonport, Moreauville and Simmsport. We finally ended up in Morganza, Louisiana, for the night at a campground. We felt good about spending a day in Cajun Country, even though the temperature was 90 degrees with high humidity.

Today's Lesson: Be proud of your family heritage and find out more about your family roots whenever possible.

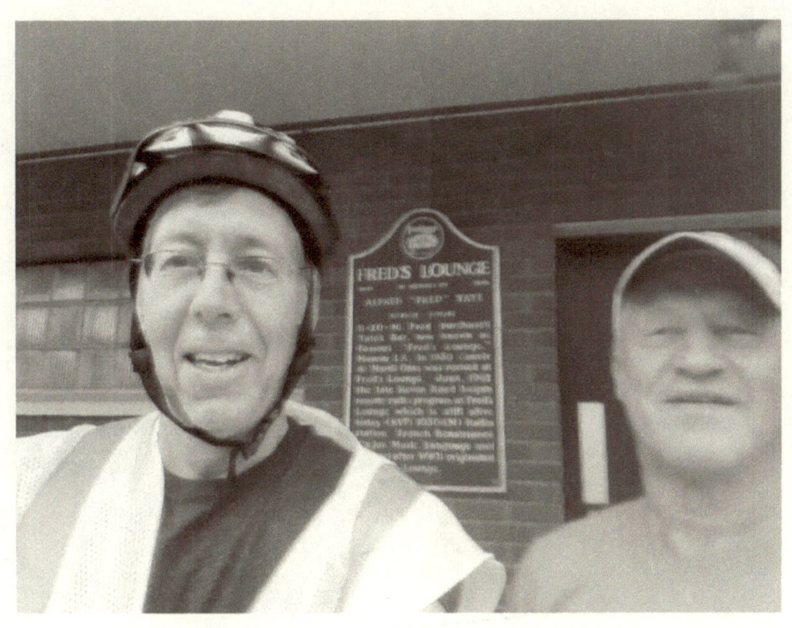

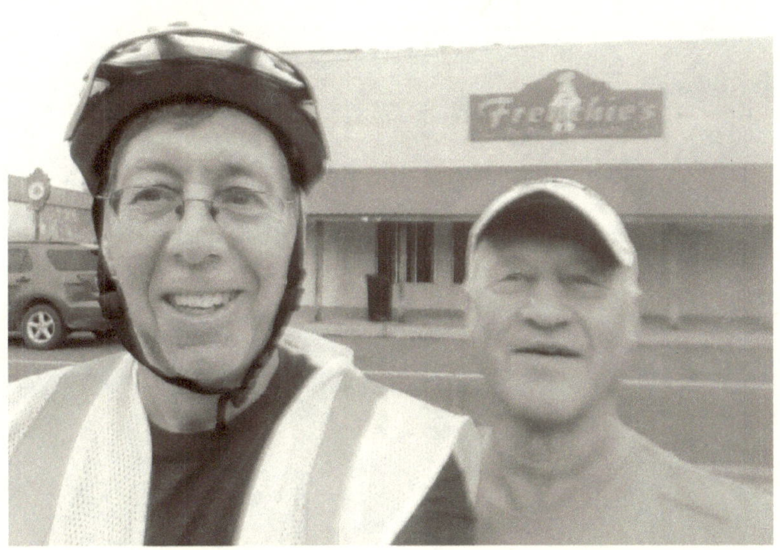

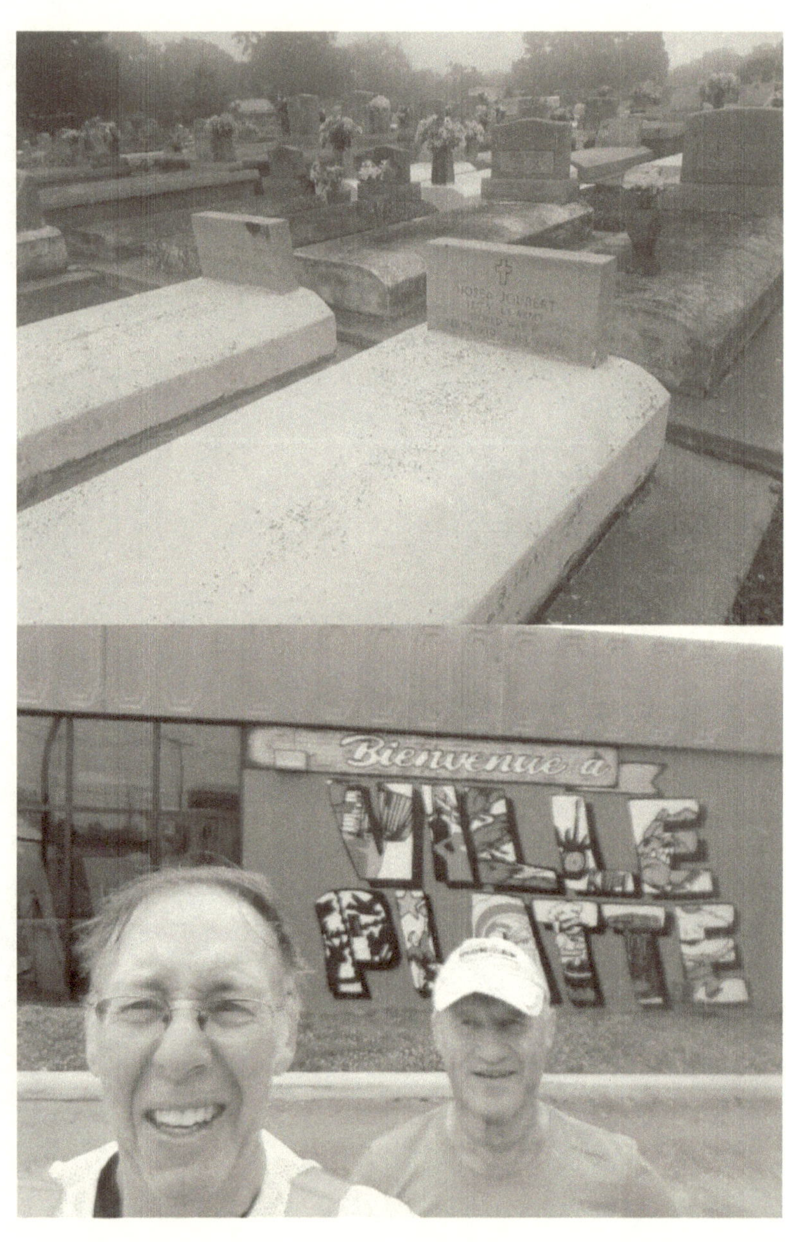
Bienvenue à
VILLE PLATTE

May 5, 2022 – Day 19 of the Bike Trip

I was the first to ride that morning out of Morganza, Louisiana. It was a sunny morning, and the daybreak was early, around 6 am. As I rode towards New Roads, Louisiana, a train ran parallel to me, about 200 feet to the right of my route. It was a long train with multiple colored train cars. The conductor blew his horn often due to the many street intersections he was crossing. This reminded me of my dad, my brother and my grandfather, who were so proud of working on the railroad during their long careers. The train was going about 15 miles an hour, relatively slow due to the traffic, which happened to be the same speed at which I was riding my bike. We rode next to each other for about 4 miles. It personally made me feel warm inside, something I cannot describe.

My ride continued through New Roads and then over a long bridge crossing the Mississippi River. I stopped in the middle of the bridge to take pictures and thought about the stories of Tom Sawyer and Huck Finn. It was looking like a great ride when suddenly I saw the camper stopped on the side of the road about one mile past the bridge. We had a flat tire on the camper! Suddenly the day had totally changed around from being a great ride to a sudden challenge. We made several calls for help only to find that my AAA insurance did not include RV coverage. So we called a towing garage that said they would come out and change our tire. Within an hour, this wonderful mechanic had changed the tire on the spot! We were grateful for his service. Now the challenge was to replace the spare tire he had used. So I went ahead with the camper while Phil started his biking segment, both heading towards Baton Rouge, Louisiana, in different directions. I was able to find a tire store near Baton Rouge. They recommended a new tire instead of using the spare since the spare tire had some dry cracks in it. One hour later, the tire was replaced with a new one. Now the challenge was to find out where Phil was located. Through many phone calls, we agreed to meet on the bike trail at the corner of Gardere and Nicholson Street. Through the technology of GPS and Google maps, we were able to meet at that exact location within 25 minutes!

By then, Phil was exhausted after riding 32 miles through the heat and city traffic of Baton Rouge. I took over the bike ride, following many giant levees that had been designed by the Army Corps of Engineers to protect the area from flooding by the mighty Mississippi River. Some of the levees were over 100 feet high! After traveling over 100 miles that day, we were now close to the downtown area of New Orleans. We stayed at a campground that night in River Ridge, Louisiana, just outside the city of New Orleans, after a very challenging day.

Total miles traveled on bike: 110 miles.

Today's Lesson: Sometimes, things can instantly change from being a perfect day to a disastrous day. During these challenges, be patient and understand that things will not always be perfect, but in the end, they will be okay. Just be patient!

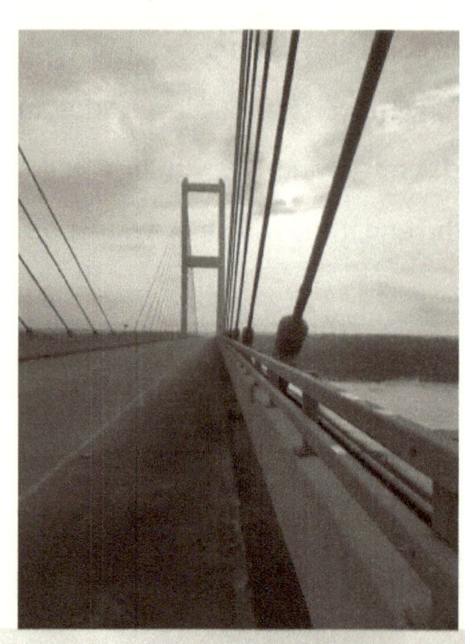

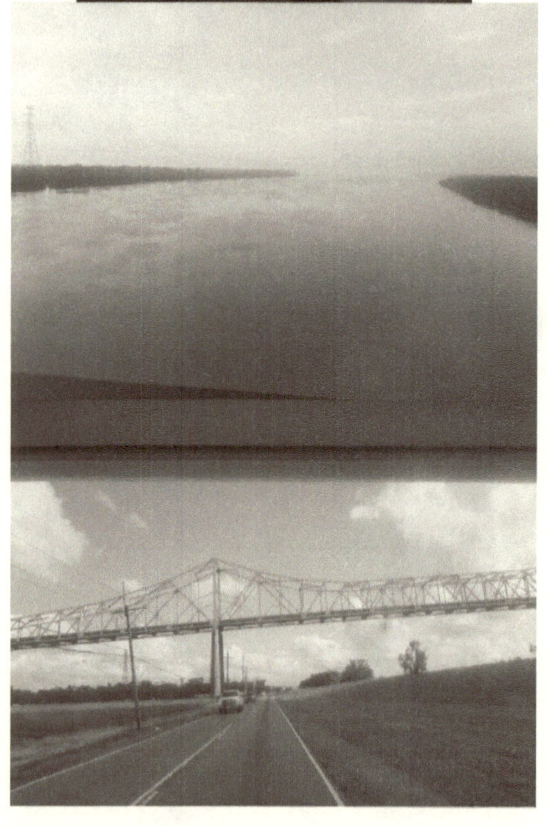

May 6, 2022 – Day 20 of the Bike Trip

Today was an unusual day for us. We knew that the weather was going to be rainy in the morning, so we decided to enjoy a partial "Day Off" from biking and enjoy some time in New Orleans. The plan was to leave the camper close to our campground and ride our bikes together into New Orleans to enjoy the sites. It turned out to work out beautifully! We started our ride by following the bike path located on top of the Levees that surround the City – (very well done) and then exited in Audubon Park, where we would take St. Charles Street all the way to the French Quarters. We even rode our bikes through Bourbon Street! Once we had visited many of the sites, we rode our bikes back the same route to our camper. We enjoyed the camaraderie of biking together for the first time on this trip! We traveled by camper to our next campsite just east of downtown New Orleans. We swam in the pool, enjoyed a good meal, and called it another great day!

Total miles traveled on bike: 60 miles.

Today's Lesson: It is good to do activities with others and share good memories together. Make sure to make good friends that you can trust and enjoy activities together.

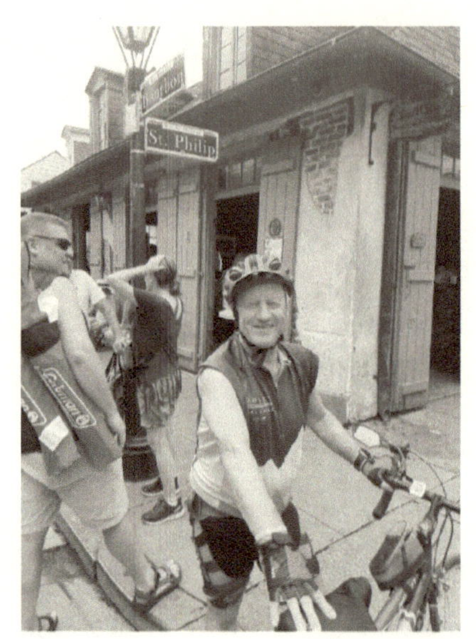

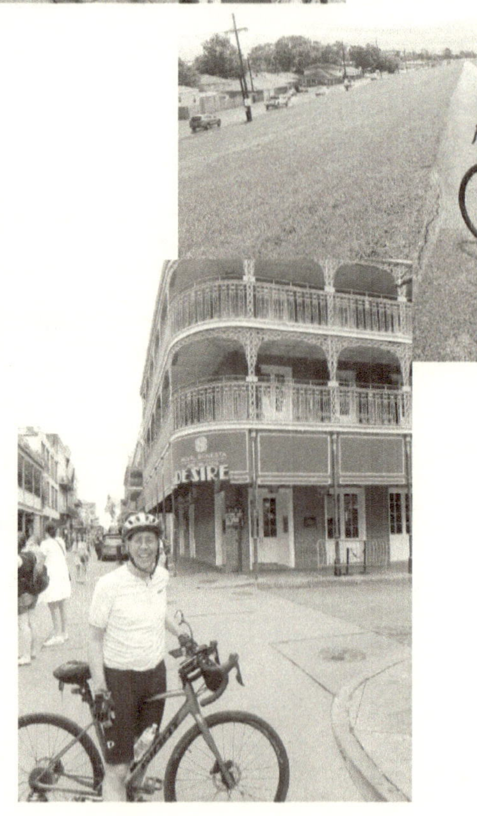

May 7, 2022 – Day 21 of the Bike Trip

We started the day just east of New Orleans and traveled Route 90 through some marshlands with clusters of vacation homes placed on stilts for foundations. We continued east until we reached the Mississippi border. We rode on a bike path that was adjacent to the beach, through the towns of Bay St. Louis, Long Beach and eventually Gulfport and Biloxi, Mississippi. The beaches were covered with fine, whitish sand. It was still early in the morning, so most of the beaches were empty. I continued biking past the many hotels and casinos in Biloxi. The day was sunny and hot. However, we had a small tailwind that really added to the speed of the ride. After two legs of 25 miles, I did not want the day to end. So we each added an additional 15 miles to our day!

By mid-afternoon, we were in Alabama, having biked in three states in one day! We were tired and hungry. We had a large meal in Mobile, Alabama and found a campground just south of Mobile, close to where we had finished today's bike ride. At the campground, we were met by a gentleman from Rockland, Maine. He had spotted our camper license plate from Maine and came over to introduce himself. It turns out that he was a retired Maine State Policeman who winters in this campground. In fact, I had done his initial medical exam when he entered the Maine State Police Academy in 1993. He reminisced about his days as a State Policeman and prior Navy Seal. Phil and I listened and thanked him for his service. We retired to our camper for an early sleep since it had been a long but very productive day.

Total miles traveled on bike: 135 miles.

Today's Lesson: No matter how far you travel, there is always a good chance that you will meet someone familiar to your past. Always make sure that your last meeting with someone is always left on a positive note.

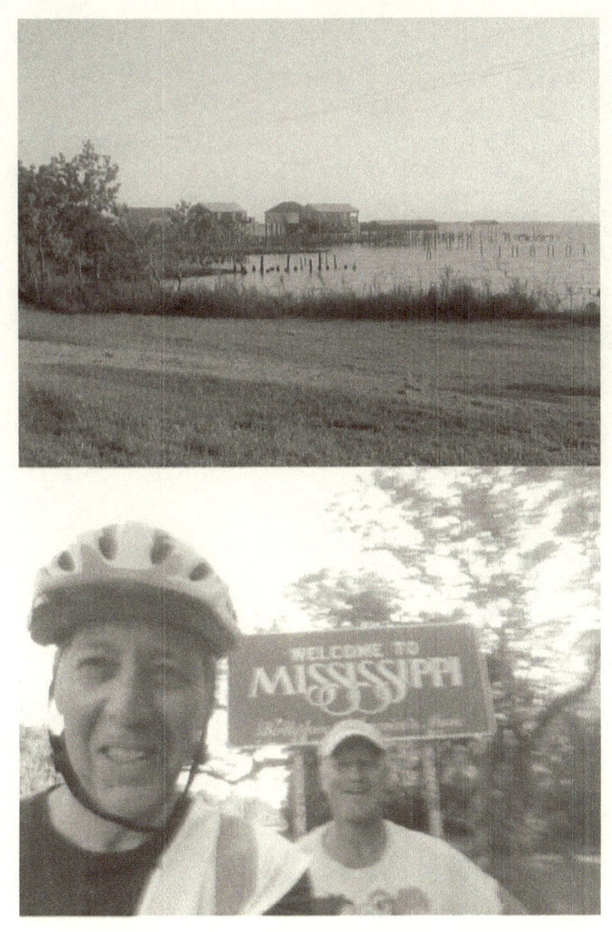

WELCOME TO
MISSISSIPPI

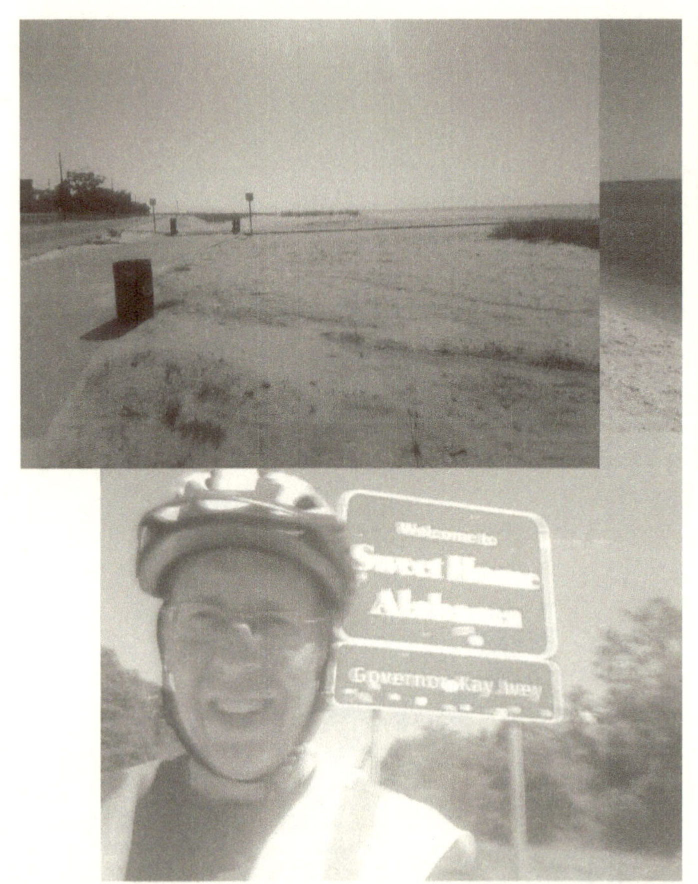
Welcome to
Sweet Home
Alabama
Governor Kay Ivey

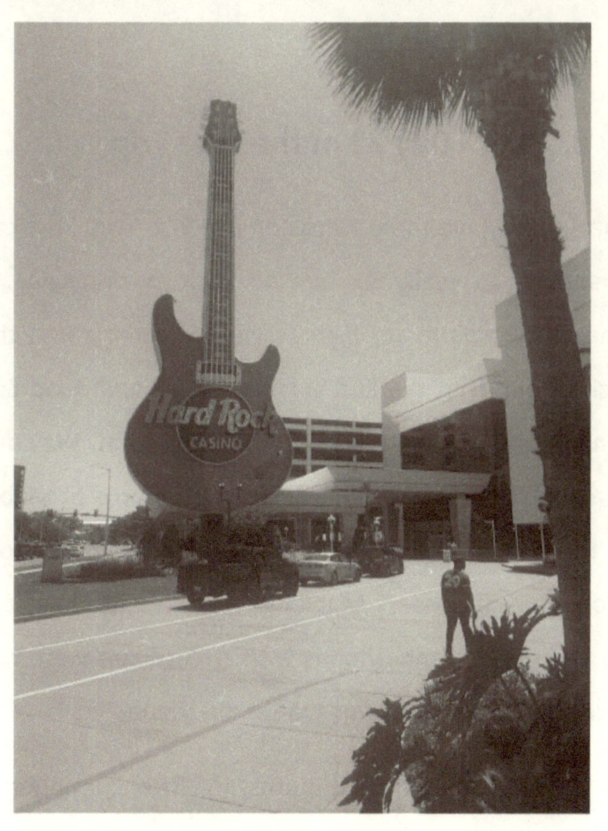

Hard Rock
CASINO

May 8, 2022 - Day 22 of the Bike Trip

We have now gone three weeks on our Bike Trip. Physically, we are holding up well. So far, no injuries or major muscle soreness. Our spirits are high as we are coming into the final stretch of our Trip! We left Mobile, Alabama, around 6:30 am, passing by the USS Alabama battleship museum. We continued over a large body of water and into the suburbs of Mobile. We rode through some beautiful small towns, such as Montrose, Fairhope, which borders Mobile Bay, and Point Clear, and into some beautiful neighborhoods with streets that were tunneled with tree branches providing wonderful shade.

Once we were out of the suburbs, the trail continued by the Alabama coastline and into a well-groomed Gulf State Park which was full of walkers and bikers. The bike path in the Park was seven miles long through windy paved paths. The route then continued to follow the beaches of the Alabama coastline and eventually onto the Florida State line. Traffic got much heavier as we approached the area of Pensacola, Florida. We were fortunate to have a well-protected road shoulder to bike on. Phil had the last section of the bike ride, which followed the outside parameter of the city of Pensacola. We each added an additional seven miles to our bike ride and ended up at a campground in Milton, Florida. We had a buffet meal at a grocery store called Piggley Wiggley. Phil was fascinated by the name and posted pictures of the store sign on Facebook. After eating on picnic tables outside of the store, we returned to our campground to play a round of mini golf. As we were playing, we heard someone call out our names! We looked up to see Bob Bouchard and his wife Collet, good friends from our hometown, who were visiting their daughter Dawn, who happened to live in Milton and had seen Phil's post on Facebook. They cleverly went looking for us at this local campground and found us. What a small world!

We sat and talked and laughed about the whole situation. After a great visit, we returned to the camper for a rest after a long hot day.

Total miles traveled on bike: 115 miles.

Today's Lesson: Social media has added a new way of communication that helps connect friends. However, the best part of communication is to sit down as a group and have a good conversation where laughter and eye-to-eye contact with each other can help us express our true feelings.

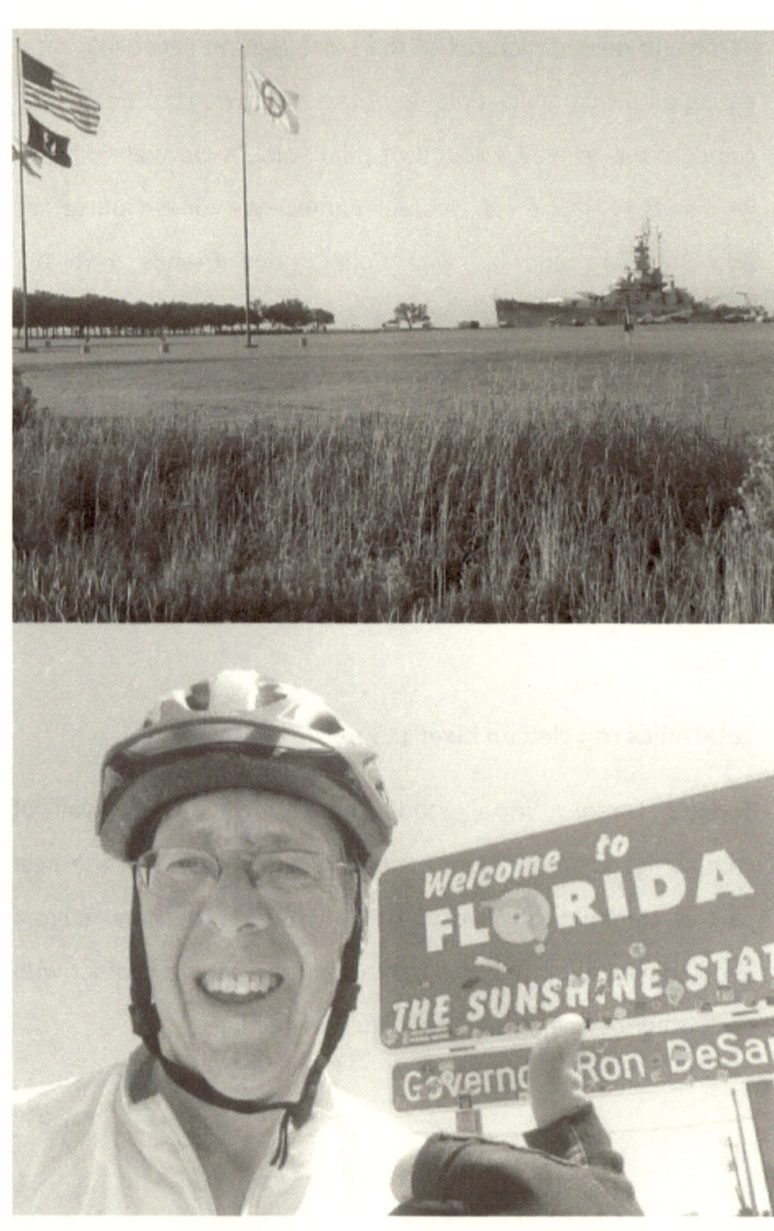

Welcome to
FLORIDA
THE SUNSHINE STAT
Governor Ron DeSa

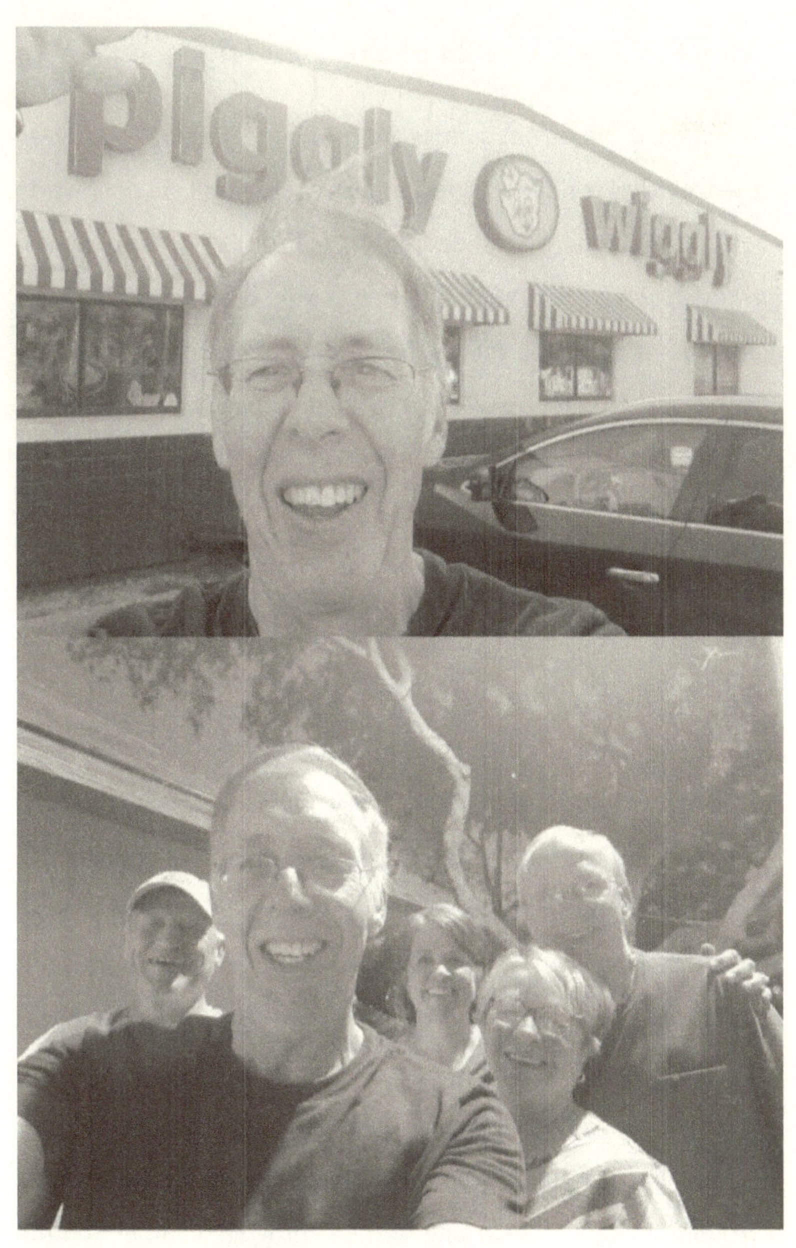
pigoly
wiggly

May 9, 2022 – Day 23 of the Bike Trip

We started the day at sunrise from Milton, Florida. Phil started the trek with a ride through the Blackwater Trail section, which was a back road that ended up on Route 90. My first leg was through some fast traffic, but with a wide bike shoulder to ride on. The terrain was mostly flat, with gentle rolling hills. The worst part of the ride was a 5 to 10-mph headwind that lasted all day. The day became hot, in the low 90's with low humidity. I did feel some dehydration at the end of my second leg and had to slow down my pace and drink more water.

We rode through the towns of Crestview, DeFuniak Springs, Ponce De Leon, Bonifay and Chipley. We ended our ride that day in Marianna, Florida, at a campground near a beautiful lake. The lady at the campground desk was extremely nice and friendly. She took our reservation and described the history of the campground that had been destroyed by hurricane Michael in 2018. She even gave us some recommendations on local restaurants that we should try for dining. Even though she was not the owner, she took pride in her job and in the campground where she worked. Her job was an excellent fit for her personality. We had a great BBQ dinner that night, took a walk around the pond area, and settled into our camper for the night. Overall, it was a very productive day.

Total miles traveled on bike: 125 miles.

Today's Lesson: It doesn't matter what you do for an occupation in life. What matters is that you do your work with commitment and dedication. Find an occupation you are passionate about, and make sure you see the purpose of the job. Always remember: Passion and Purpose are important to make you happy with your job.

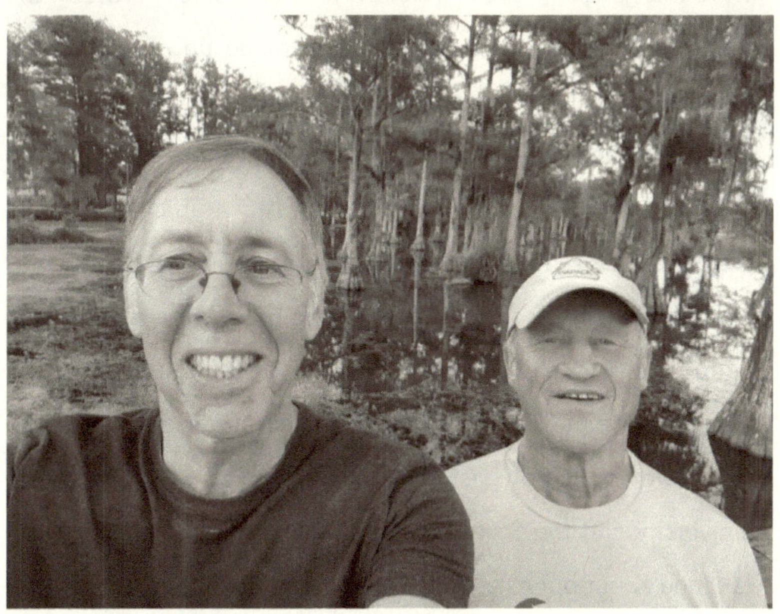

May 10, 2022 – Day 24 of the Bike Trip

It was another beautiful sunny day in northern Florida. I began the first leg of the bike ride, starting in Marianna, Florida, at dawn. The road quickly went into some back roads with very little traffic. I had the whole road to myself!

The road had gentle hills which were easy to climb, and the wind was gentle. There were a few fenced-in cattle farms on the way. However, most of the trail was made up of a beautiful wooded area. We rode in rural areas past the towns of Chattahoochee, Quincy, and Midway until we got to Tallahassee, Florida. At that time, the traffic picked up tremendously (and so did the route confusion). The bike lanes through the city were very narrow, and there were many traffic lights. It was a challenge for the bike rider (me) and for the camper driver (Phil). After many missed street signs and one ways, we finally got past the city after going by Florida State University and the State Capital building. Afterward, Phil and I laughed about our experience of going through the city.

Good friends can find humor in stressful situations. That is why you can support each other through some tough times. We have known each other for years and have strong trust and support for each other. Sure, we sometimes have our differences of opinions and sometimes need our space alone.

However, we both know that without each other's support, this trip would not be possible. Neither one of us could have made this trip alone. But together, we are stronger and can achieve our goal! We continued our trip on Route 90 past small towns such as Chaires, Monticello, and Greenville. We ended the day in Madison, Florida, at a wonderful campground located on a golf course. We had dinner at a Bistro in Madison and then went site seeing in town. It was a beautiful small town with unique architecture. We ended the day relaxing at the campground and preparing for tomorrow's journey.

Total miles traveled on bike: 125 miles.

Today's Lesson: Friends are a gift. Supporting each other through challenges makes things that seem overwhelming become possibilities. Sharing adventures with a friend or loved one makes it much more enjoyable. Respect your friends. They may not be perfect, but neither are you.

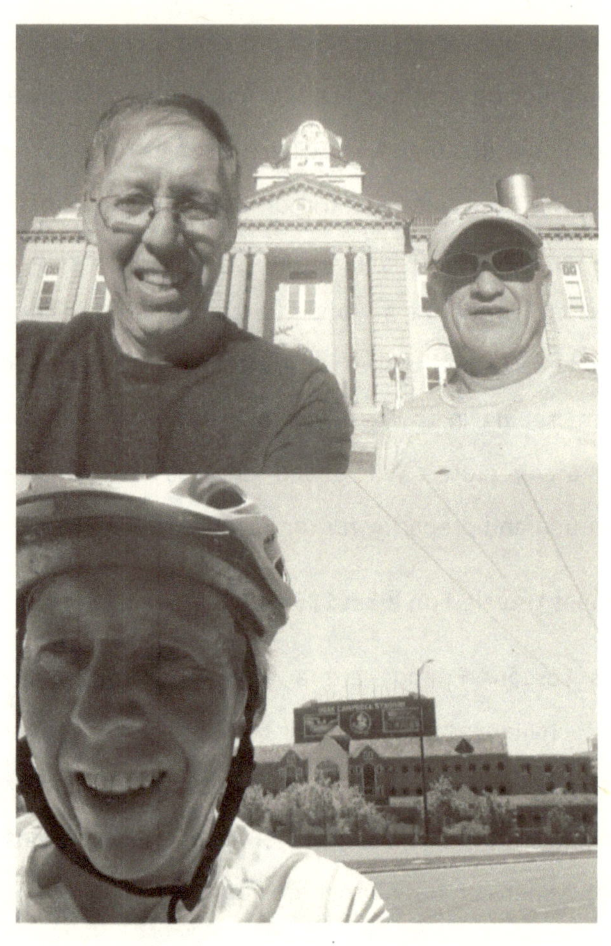

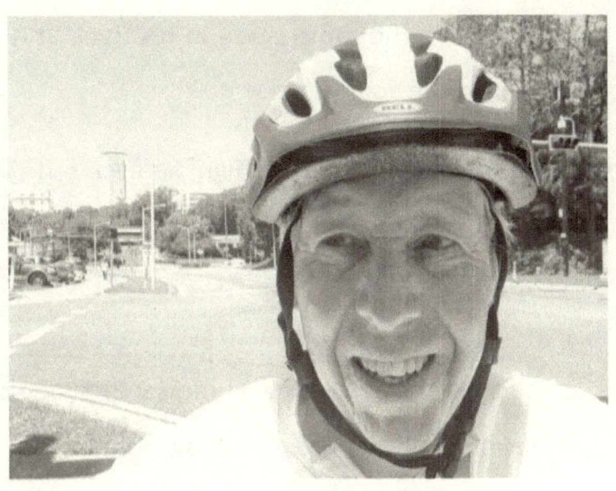

May 11, 2022 – Day 25 of the Bike Trip

The day started early out of Madison, Florida. Conditions were perfect; cool morning start with bright sunshine during the day and temperature in the 80s. The road conditions were also ideal, with well-paved back roads, very little traffic and a tailwind. We continued following our GPS maps, passing by small cattle farms and plenty of wooded areas. At one exchange, I was resting in the camper on the side of the road when a large dump truck stopped behind me. He was checking to see if we needed help with the camper. I assured him that we were okay. He then asked what part of Maine we were from. (He had seen our Maine license plate). He stated that he was also from Maine, having graduated high school from Dover-Foxcroft in 1982. He moved to Florida at age 37 and bought a house by the Suwanee River. We had a nice conversation about life in Maine, and then he drove away in his truck. It is always nice to see people from your home state.

We continued past the towns of High Springs and Alachua, ending the day just north of Gainesville, Florida. Phil had been corresponding with some golfing friends from the St. John Valley that wintered in Ocala, Florida. They wanted to see us on our trip. So the three friends met us at our campground outside of Gainesville, where we went to a seafood restaurant in Starks, Florida. We had a good visit with them, talking about our trip and sharing memories of the "Valley." Our day had been complete after traveling over 100 miles through some beautiful areas of northern Florida in record time. During the day's ride, we had also seen seven other bikers in full saddle gear who were riding together with the same destination – Southern Tier bike ride across the United States. We were all close to the end of our ride, and we knew it. It was a mixed feeling of relief while not wanting this experience to end! We settled quietly that night, knowing we had experienced one of the best rides of our trip due to the ideal conditions. Life was good!

Total miles traveled on bike: 125 miles.

Today's Lesson: It is always wonderful to meet people from your home State when you are traveling. It always seems comforting when you can share something in common. No matter where you are traveling, there is always a connection somewhere with your roots. Be proud of your hometown and State.

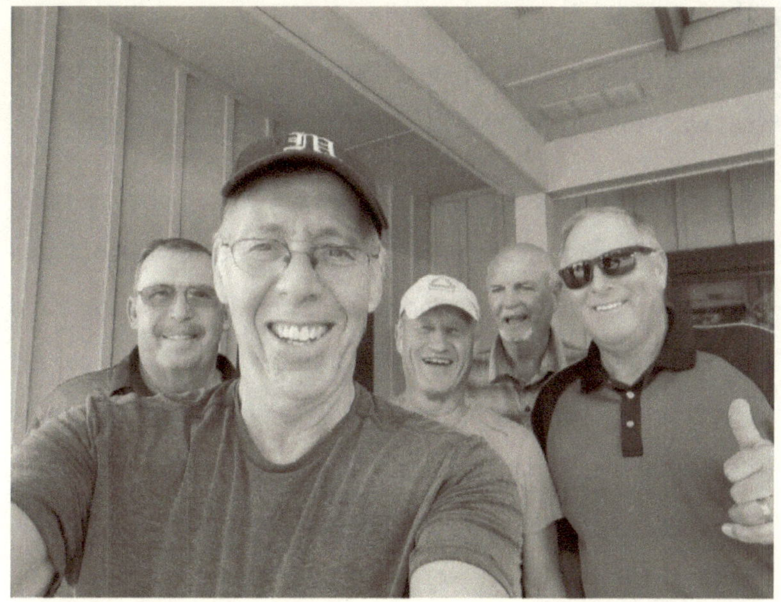

May 12, 2022 – Day 26 of the Bike Trip

We knew that this would be our last biking day on this trip. This was it! After 25 days of biking, it had all come down to this day. The ride was going to be emotional. Part of us wanted the trip to be over, as our bodies were tired. The other part of us did not want this to end.

We took off on a bike trail north of Gainesville, Florida. Despite much traffic on the road next to the trail, we quickly went into a city park that was very secluded, surrounded only by trees and wildlife. This bike trail seemed to go on forever! It was a perfect conclusion to our ride. On the path, we went through the towns of Hawthorne, Florahome and Palatka. We also rode through Hastings, Florida, which is the potato-growing capital of Florida. Next to the bike trails were many potato fields ready to be harvested. As I approached a large farm, there was a potato harvester in the field, cultivating their crop from the sandy soil. It reminded me of my youth when we had to wake up early in the morning to pick potatoes for farmers in the fall. In those days, our school would close for four weeks, as local farmers would hire school children to pick the potatoes. We would be paid 25 cents per barrel picked. We would usually pick between 50 to 100 barrels a day. It was hard work at that young age. However, it taught us the value of hard work, a lesson we never forgot. As I passed that harvester today, it seemed like my work life had come full circle. It was comforting.

We arrived in St. Augustine in the early afternoon after completing nearly 100 miles under partly cloudy skies but comfortable temperatures in the 70s. The city was filled with people as we rode into town together. We came to our final destination, the Bridge of Lions! There were many "high-fives" and pictures taken. We had made it! We went to St. Augustine beach and brought our bike tires into the Atlantic Ocean, completing the trip from coast to coast. It was a perfect ending to a perfect trip!

That evening, we took a guided tour of the city of St. Augustine, experiencing all of the sites and history of this ancient city. We then met a relative of Phil's at a very nice restaurant, where he treated us to a wonderful meal. We then retired to our campground, which was soon followed by a good night's sleep.

Our goal was accomplished! It had been a long and challenging trip. However, it was so gratifying and rewarding to know that we had completed our initial goal. My bucket list item had been fulfilled!

Total miles traveled on bike: 105 miles

Today's Lesson: Hold close your dreams. With hard work, you can accomplish what some people think is impossible. Anything is possible if you want it bad enough and work hard.

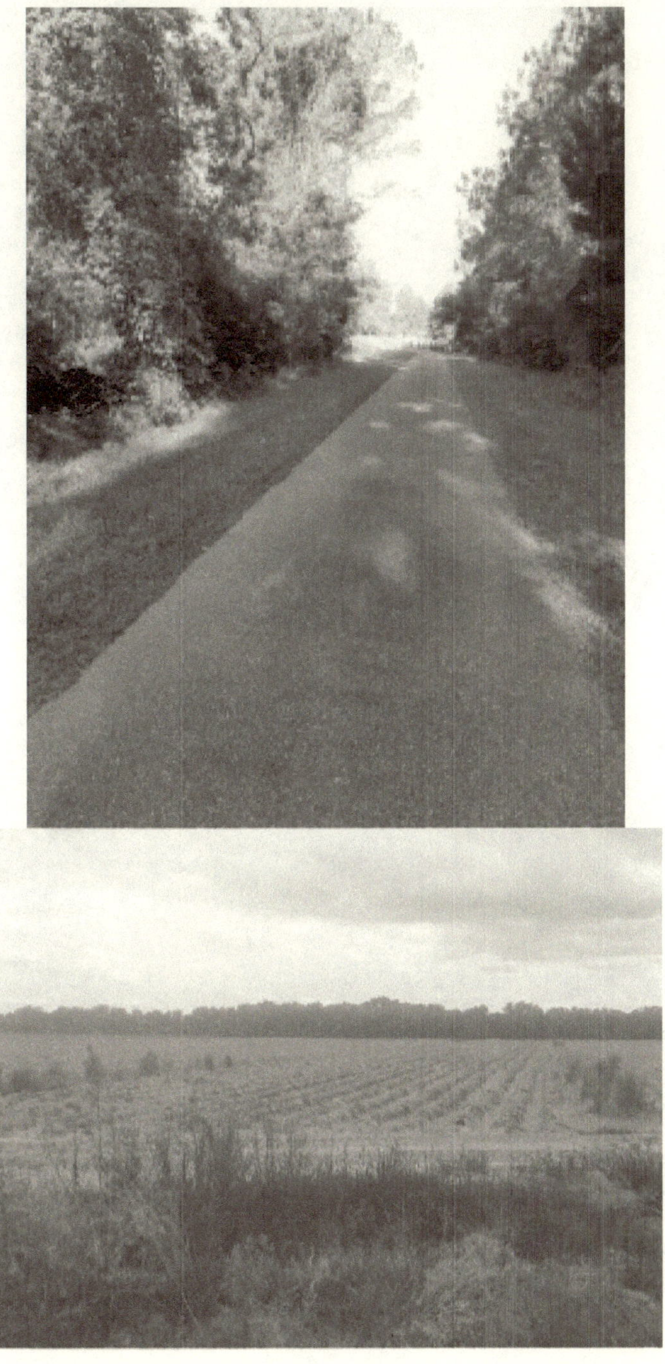

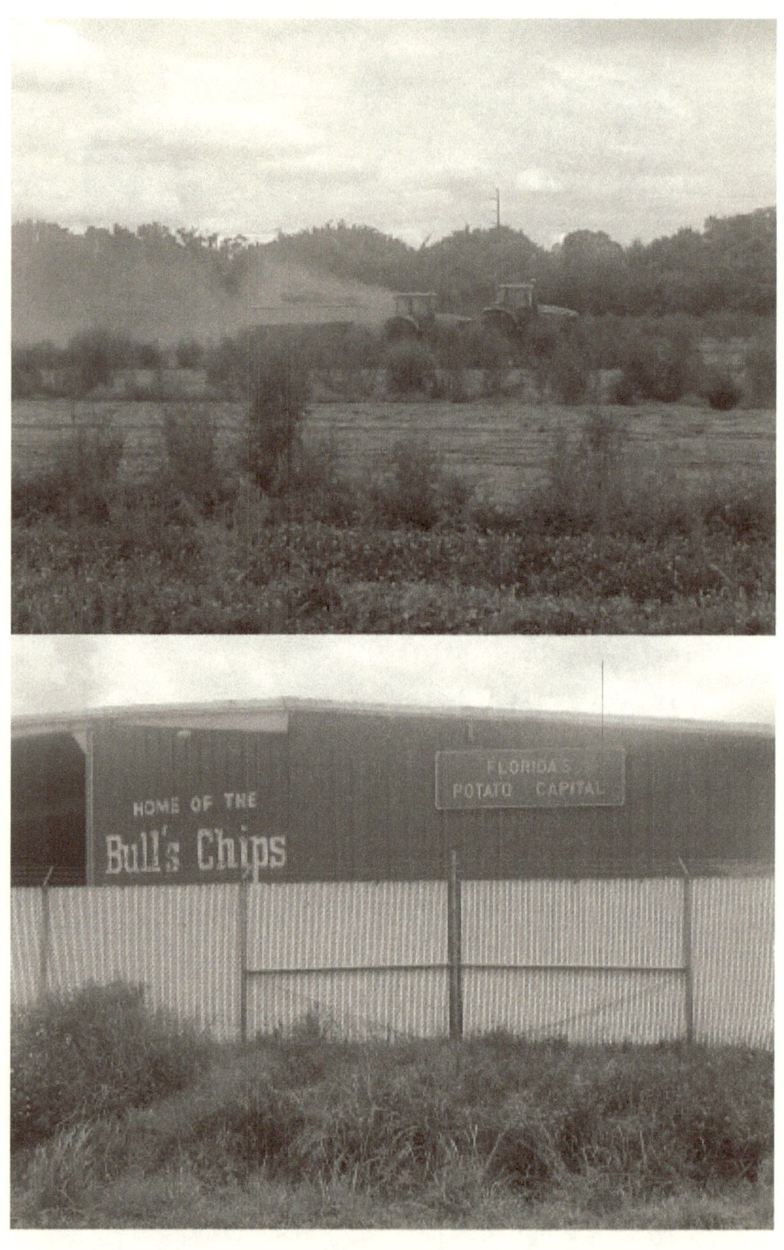
HOME OF THE
Bull's Chips
FLORIDA'S
POTATO CAPITAL

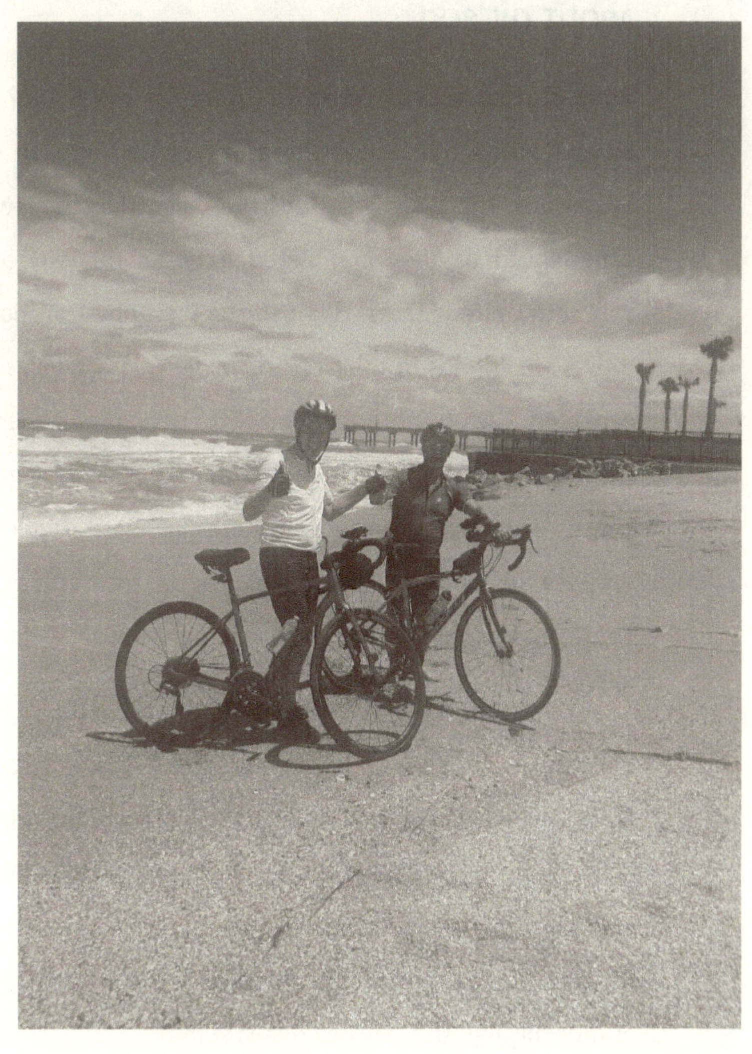

ABOUT THE BOOK:

What started as a "bucket list" item for the author to ride a bicycle across the United States developed into an incredible adventure. The book describes the daily trials that two friends experienced as they completed a two-man relay across the southern United States. What started as a physical challenge for these two friends in their 60s developed into much more than expected. Each day brought daily experiences of life lessons that we take for granted and need to share with a new generation. These experiences include friendship, hard work, passion, purpose, patience, understanding, caring, trust and many more. These lessons are described in detail with each daily journal entry.

The book is designed to inspire readers of all ages to accomplish lifetime adventures that they never thought possible. It will challenge you to reflect on the important things in life to share with your children and grandchildren. Each daily journal will also describe the true beauty of this wonderful country. Follow the author through this journey of a lifetime!